INTERMITTENT FASTING FOR WOMEN & KETOGENIC DIET FOR WOMEN

VIRGINIA COOKE

© Copyright 2020 by Virginia Cooke

All rights reserved.

This book is driven towards providing reliable information towards a better way of living. The publication is sold such that the publisher is not required to offer officially permitted or qualified services. For advice, either professional or legal, you can contact a practiced individual in the profession.

Under no condition should this document be duplicated, reproduced, or transmitted in any printed format or by any electronic means. Any storage or recording of this document is not allowed unless with written permission from the publisher.

The information provided here is therefore stated to be truthful, and consistent and any liability in terms of abuse of policies or inattention is the sole responsibility of the reader. No legal blame or responsibility can be held against the publisher for any damages or monetary loss due to the information provided here, directly or indirectly.

The information provided herein is solely offered for informational purposes, and the presentation of the data is without any guaranteed assurance or contract.

Trademarks used are without any consent, and the publication of the trademark is without permission and backing by the owner of the trademark. The trademarks used in this book are for descriptive purposes only and are owned by people not affiliated to with this book.

INTRODUCTION

Imagine a scenario in which I can reveal to you how to eat your way skinny. You'd most likely think I was insane or expected it had something to do with ingesting spaghetti produced from tapeworms. In any case, you'd not be right. The fact is there is a way that you could eat your way to significant and long term fat loss results. It's called ketogenics.

Ketogenics is a term that basically required your body to enter a state called ketosis. The body generally makes use of carbohydrate as its primary source of energy. This owes to the fact that carbohydrates are the easiest for the body to absorb. Ketosis occurs when your body begins using fat as its main source of energy above all other types of energy sources including proteins and carbohydrates. Once your body enters this state it becomes much easier for your body to utilize stored fat deposits for energy thus resulting in automatic and ongoing fat loss.

Be that as it may, if the body run out of carbohydrates, it reverts to making use of fats and protein for its energy production. Essentially, the body has a sort of energy hierarchy which it follows. Right off the bat, the body is modified to utilize carbohydrate as as energy fuel when it is available. Secondly, it will revert to using fats as an alternative in the absence of an adequate supply of carbohydrate.

Finally, the body convert proteins for its vitality arrangement in when there is an extraordinary consumption of its sugar and fat stores. However, breaking down proteins for energy provision leads to a general loss of lean muscle mass.

The ketogenic diet doesn't completely rely upon the calories. This is because the composition of those calories matters because of the hormonal reaction of the body to various macronutrients.

In any case, there are two schools of thought in the keto community. While one believes that the amount of calories and fat consumption does not matter, the other contends that calories and fat does matter.

When using a ketogenic diet, you are attempting a discovery parity point. While calories matter, the creation of those calories also counts. In a ketogenic diet, the most significant factor of the composition of those calories is the balance of fat, protein and carbohydrates and how each affects insulin levels. This balance is very important because any rise in insulin will stop lipolysis. Therefore, you need to eat foods that will surely create the minimum rise in insulin. This will help you keep your body in the state of burning stored body fat for fuel. The body can usually go into a ketosis state. This is often the case when you are in a fasting state such as when you are asleep. In this state, the body tends to burn fats for energy while the body carries out its repairs and growth while you are sleeping.

Carbohydrates generally make up most of the calories in a regular meal. As well, the body is inclined to make use of the carbohydrate as energy as it is more easily absorbable. The proteins and fats in the diet are thus more likely to be stored. However, in a ketogenic diet, most of the calories come from fats rather than carbohydrates itself. Since ketogenic diets have a low amount of carbohydrates, they are immediately used up. The low carbohydrate level causes an apparent shortage of energy fuel for the body. As a result of this seeming shortage, the body resorts to its stored fat content. It makes a shift from a carbohydrate-consumer to a fat-burner. The body however, does not make use of the fats in the recently ingested meal but rather stores them up for the next round of ketosis. As the body gets more familiar to burning fat for energy, fats in an ingested meal become used up with little left for storage.

This is why the ketogenic diet uses a high amount of fat consumption so that the body can have enough for energy production and also still be able to store enough fat. The body needs to be able to store some fat otherwise it will start breaking down its protein stores in muscles during the ketosis period. In fasting periods for example, during ketosis, in between dinners and during sleep, the body still needs a steady supply of energy. You have these periods in your day and so you have to expend enough measures of fat for your body to use as energy. If there are no adequate amounts of stored fat, the proteins contained in your muscle become the next option for the body to use as energy. It is therefore important to eat enough to avoid this scenario from taking place. The main goal of a ketogenic diet is to mimic the state of starvation in the body. Ketogenic diets deprive the body of its preferred immediate and easily convertible carbohydrates by restricting and severely cutting back on carbohydrate intake. This situation forces it into a fat-burning mode for energy production.

Things being what they are, if ketogenics is so staggering and can be your response to fat why haven't you heard of it? Well, you probably have. Ketosis is at the core of many fat loss programs and diets including the incredibly popular Atkins program. Some people fear this diet because it touts ingesting large amounts of fatty foods which some believe could be extremely harmful to your body. The fact of the matter is that when your body enters the state of ketosis it will burn most if not all of these fats for energy so very little will be stored in the body or broken down and result in fat in the blood stream. To comprehend why this ketogenic diet can be so viable at burning fat you need to take a look at how your body typically works. The body's preferred source of fuel is carbohydrates and is very effective at metabolizing carbohydrates to use for fuel. Because of this fact, your body actually craves carbohydrates on a regular basis which usually leads to us over eating them. At a point when the body eats too many carbohydrates than it can process and use, it separates them, converts them and stores some of them as fat for later use. But in case your body does not have a source of carbohydrates to use for vitality, it will use the next accessible source. If you seriously limit the amount of carbohydrates that you eat and rather replace it with fat, your body will go through a process and adjustment that will allow it to metabolize the fat for energy as well. In addition, when the body starts to utilize fat as fuel it will be much easier for it to metabolize stored fat as fuel thereby helping to speed up existing fat loss. The ketogenic diet was widely used for the next several decades in treating epilepsy both in children and adults. In several epilepsy studies, about 50% of patients reported having at least 50% reduction in seizures. In as much as the arrival of anticonvulsant drugs in the 1940s and afterwards relegated the ketogenic diet to an "alternative" medicine. Most health center givers, as well as patients, found it a lot easier to use the pills as well as adhering to the strict ketogenic diet. It was subsequently ignored in the treatment of epilepsy by most specialists.

In the year 1993, a renewed interest in the ketogenic diet was ignited by Hollywood producer Jim Abrahams by name. Abraham had his two years old son, Charlie, brought to the Johns Hopkins Hospital for epilepsy treatment. Charlie experienced rapid seizure control within days of using ketogenic diet. Jim, Charlie's father creates the Charlie Foundation which helped to revive research efforts. His production of a TV movie called "First Do No Harm" starring Meryl Streep really helped to massively promote the ketogenic diet. The meals were designed to provide the body with the right amount of protein it needs for growth and repair. The calculation of the amount of used calories was done to provide suitable amounts that will be able to support and maintain the proper weight necessary for the child's height and weight.

Increased healthy fat consumption is the main focus of the ketogenic diet. Also, the purpose is to maintain the state of ketosis at all times thus allowing your body to use more body fat for fuel. The body digests fat and protein differently. Fat is arguably the body's best source of energy and in a state of ketosis, the body can make use of body fat and dietary fat equally well. In general, fats have a very limited effect on blood sugar levels and insulin production in your body. However, protein affects both of these levels if consumed in large amounts beyond what your body requires. When using a ketogenic diet, your body becomes more of a fat-burner than a carbohydrate-dependent machine. Many researches have linked the consumption of increased amounts of carbohydrates to the development of many illnesses such as diabetes and insulin resistance. By nature, carbohydrates are simply absorbable and therefore can also be stored easily by the body. Digestion of carbohydrates starts right from the moment you put them into your mouth. As soon as you begin chewing them, amylase (the enzymes that digest carbohydrate) in your saliva is already acting on the carbohydrate-containing food.

In the stomach, carbohydrates are broken down. When they get into the small intestines, they are then absorbed into the bloodstream. On getting to the bloodstream, carbohydrates in general increase the blood sugar level. This increase in blood sugar level stimulates the immediate release of insulin into the bloodstream. The higher the increase in blood sugar levels, the more the amount of insulin that is unconfined. Insulin is a hormone that causes excess sugar in the bloodstream to be removed in order to lower the blood sugar level. Insulin takes the sugar and carbohydrate that you eat and stores them either as glycogen in muscle tissues or as fat in adipose tissue for future use as energy. However, the body can develop what is known as insulin resistance when it is constantly exposed to such high amounts of glucose in the bloodstream. This scenario can easily cause obesity as the body tends to quickly store any excess amount of glucose. Health conditions, such as diabetes and cardiovascular disease can also a result from this situation. Keto diets are low in carbohydrate and high in fat and have been associated with reducing and improving many health conditions.

One of the foremost things a ketogenic diet does is to stabilize your insulin levels and also restore leptin signaling. The paramount part of the diet is to prompt the body to consume fat rather than carbohydrate, which has the effect of fast weight loss. The high-fat content can cause surprise and worry in a health-conscious society which associates 'fat' with 'bad.' However, great fats are healthy and essential as part of a controlled and balanced diet. Escalated levels of carbohydrates, on the other hand, can cause a spike in glycogen levels, which can lead to stoutness and low energy levels. Part of the intrigue is the ketogenic diet is its success in achieving quick weight loss, so it is ideal for those with many pounds to shed. The diet excludes high carbohydrate foods such as starchy fruits and vegetables, bread, pasta and sugar while increasing high fat foods such as cream and butter. A typical meal might include fish or chicken with green vegetables, followed by fruit with lots of cream. Breakfast might be bacon and eggs, a snack cheese with cucumber. There are many variants of the diet which including more relaxed versions of the regime. The initial few days of a ketogenic diet involves the body adapting to a different way of eating, which can prompt a feeling of 'withdrawal'. This is no surprise as modern western diet and foods are heavy in starch and sugar. Following this adaptation period, however, those eating a ketogenic diet begin to enjoy many benefits. In addition to fast weight loss, there are increased energy levels. The ketogenic diet can also be very enjoyable, with delicious fish, steaks, bacon, eggs and fruit with cream on the menu. Enjoyment of food is important if the diet is to prove sustainable.

TABLE OF CONTENTS

INTERMITTENT FASTING FOR WOMEN 1

Foreword 3
Preface 4
Chapter 1 – The Science Of The Female Body And The Difficulty In Weight Loss 5
    Women Have A Lean Body Mass 5

Chapter 2 – The Basics Of Intermittent Fasting For Women 9
    What Is Intermittent Fasting? 9
    Why Intermittent Fasting 10
    Differences Between Intermittent Fasting In Men And Women 11
    What Are Calories? 12
    Health Benefits Of Intermittent Fasting For Women 12

Chapter 3 – Types Of Intermittent Fasting For Women 17
    Side Effects And Safety Of Intermittent Fasting 19
    How Intermittent Fasting Affects Your Cells And Hormones As A Woman 21
    Can You Practice A Quick Workout While On A Fast? 22
    How Can You Practice Fasting Safely? 25
    Intermittent Fasting Tips For Beginners 27

Chapter 4 – Types Of Weight Loss Diet Plans 31
    The Paleo Diet 31

The Vegan Diet 32
The Keto Diet 34
The Dukan Diet 35
The Ultra-Low-Fat Diet 37
The Atkins Diet 38
The Hcg Diet 40
The Zone Diet 41
What Is The Keto Diet? 43
Benefits Of The Ketogenic Diet 44
How To Use Intermittent Fasting On The Keto Diet 48
Benefits Of Intermittent Fasting On The Keto Diet 49
Who Shouldn't Practice Intermittent Fasting On A Keto Diet? 51
The Reason Why Our Keto Diet Differs From Other Keto Diets 52
14- Days Keto Diet Meal Plan And Recipes On Intermittent Fasting 57
Shopping List 57
Shopping List 72

Chapter 5 - Keto Cook Book For Intermittent Fasting. 83

Day 1 83
Day 2 91
Day3 99
Day4 106
Day5 114
Day6 122
Day7 130
Day 8 137
Day9 146
Day10 153
Day11 161
Day12 168

Day 13 175
Day14 183
Day15 188
Day16 195
Day17 203
Day18 211
Day19 219
Day20 226
Day21 234

Faqs 241

KETOGENIC DIET FOR WOMEN 247

Preface 248
Chapter 1: General Understanding Of Ketogenic Diet
.... 250
   What Is Ketosis? 250
   What Is A Ketogenic Diet? 252
   Various Types Of Ketogenic Diets 254
   Other Health Benefits Of Keto 255
   Instructions To Eat Keto 256
   Nourishments To Avoid 256
   Nourishments To Eat 257

A Ketogenic Diet For Women 259
   Types Of Keto Diet For Women 259

Why Do Women Practice The Keto Diet 262
Chapter 2 Significant Health Benefits Of A Ketogenic Diet For Woman 264
   Regular Ketogenic Diet Mistakes For Ladies 269

The Ketogenic Diet Is Not Stressful 272
Is Keto Good For Women? 273
Ketogenic Diet Cautions For Ladies/Women 273
Step By Step Guidelines To Get Started With A
Ketogenic Diet For Women 276
Getting Into Ketosis 276
How The Keto Diet Works For Different Women. 278
Women Who Can Benefit From A Ketogenic Diet?
.... 279
What A Ketogenic Diet Can Do To Your
Periods/Menstrual Cycle 283
Precautions To Take Before Starting Keto For Ladies
.... 287

Chapter 3 Intermittent Fasting And Keto Diet 289

What Is Intermittent Fasting? Clarified In Human
Terms 289
What Is Intermittent Fasting? 291

Intermittent Fasting For Women 310

Intermittent Fasting Affects Women Differently ... 311
Health Benefits Of Intermittent Fasting For Women
.... 312
Other Health Benefits... 315
Best Types Of Intermittent Fasting For Women 316
Safety And Side Effects 319

Keto Diet And Intermittent Fasting In-Depth 321

Strategies For Combining Intermittent Fasting With
Keto 327
Starting A Keto, Intermittent And Hybrid Fasting
Diet 336

Chapter 4- A 14-Days Ketogenic Meal Plan For Women 339

Chapter 5- Keto For Women Recipes 372

INTERMITTENT FASTING FOR WOMEN

The Complete Guide to Heal Your Body and Lose Weight Quickly and Easily Through the Process of Metabolic Autophagy

Virginia Cooke

DISCLAIMER

All information contained in this book is provided for educational and informational purposes only. The author is, therefore, not in any way accountable for any improper use of the information form this material. The information provided is useful and accurate, but the author is not bound for the proper or improper use of the information contained therein.

FOREWORD

I want to thank you for trusting me by deciding to purchase this life-transforming eBook. Thanks for spending your time and resources on this material.

I can assure you will obtain exact results if you will diligently follow the blueprint laid out in the information manual you are currently reading. It has transformed lives, and I firmly believe it will equally change your own life too.

All the information presented in this Do It Yourself piece is designed to be easy to digest and practice.

PREFACE

Congratulations on downloading my book Intermittent Fasting for Women: The Complete Guide to Heal Your Body and Lose Weight Quickly and Easily Through the Process of Metabolic Autophagy (Intermittent Fasting for Beginners). What if I told you that breakfast being the most important meal of the day was wrong? What if I told you it is more important when you eat than what you eat? Perhaps much of the nutritional dogma that we've been raised with is now outdated, like snacking all day long and eating many meals. Throughout this book, I plan to discuss with you what I believe to be the most profoundly transformational concept and strategy as it pertains to Health and Aging. Over the last 20 years, I've seen tremendous shifts in health and wellness, escalated rates of obesity, diabetes, and cardiovascular disease, many of which are preventable.

I feel so passionately about this because it's something that would benefit every woman out there. Join me as we move through the pages of *Intermittent Fasting for Women*.

CHAPTER 1 – THE SCIENCE OF THE FEMALE BODY AND THE DIFFICULTY IN WEIGHT LOSS

Weight loss is not the same when it comes to men and their female counterparts. If a man and a woman go on a weight loss adventure, the signs of weight loss begin to appear faster in men than in women. For a woman who wants to lose weight, she has to understand one thing, and that is the fact that weight loss is not something that would come easy. It is not impossible, though, but it would need consistency and the right information for things to go the right way.

You have to understand that it is not just about you and that this is a general problem all women face at the moment. There are many scientific reasons why it is harder for women to lose weight and the understanding of this difficulty, would help you in your quest to lose weight.

Women have a lean body mass

Women naturally do not have as much muscle as men do, and muscles help us burn calories better. With this in mind, knowing fully well that the availability of a larger muscle mass in men gives them a higher basal metabolic rate. Even without exercise, the male body burns more calories daily than women, leading to weight loss.

Women have less testosterone than men

The availability of more testosterone in men is another primary reason why men lose weight faster than women. With men having up to seven times more testosterone than women on average, men can build muscles a lot more than women which as we said earlier, is an excellent way to burn more calories and lose more weight in the process.

Hormonal fluctuations

The fluctuations in female hormones is something that goes from one point to another without any particular solution per time. From mid-cycle to after the monthly period, water retention is a factor. Pre-menopausal women have fluctuations in progesterone and estrogen levels leading to cycles of water loss and retention. This is a factor when it comes to weight loss and has a lot to do when it comes to how much weight can be lost and gained within these cycles.

Women store fat in a different way

The female body keeps certain types of fat and is unwilling to give it up amidst different diets and exercise sessions. The female body has been designed to at a certain point in life nourish another life, and it knows it. So before that time, the body tends to store some fat which it would not let go of easily even with some weight loss plans. A woman's body has it in mind to keep in enough body fat to produce enough Leptin for fertility and enough DHA in the lower body to build a good and healthy baby brain.

Women process and burn fat differently

When it comes to weight loss, men lose weight depending on how they workout. However, for women, it is quite different. Women lose the upper body weight first and then the lower body weight as they persist. The funny thing is that when women are pregnant, women store omega-3 fatty acid DHA in their thighs as it is an important factor for baby development. The point is simple, as a woman, and depending on whatever position you find yourself; you might find different body parts not easily giving up fat when you try to burn fat.

Differences in food preferences

This is where we say; women are the cause of their problems. Women crave high-fat foods than men. Even when women say they are not hungry, whenever they are asked to taste a cake, pizza, or chocolate stick, there is a part of the brain that triggers women to feel hungrier than they were feeling before, causing them to eat whatever it is they did not want to eat in the end.

Workout Habits

We all know where this is headed; again, this has to do with muscle mass. Women stick to cardiovascular exercises as they ought to, which does not allow them to amass enough muscles to help with weight loss and calorie consumption. To burn fat, women need to incorporate light weight lifting with their other workout routines.

Post-workout hunger hormone

Compared to men, women have a tendency to eat more after a workout. A hormone known as "ghrelin" which tells you that you are hungry, rises after women workout. The hormone known as Leptin which gives you a sense of fullness drops significantly in the process as well. Simply said, women want to eat almost immediately they workout, which is just like emptying a bucket and filling it up almost immediately.

Emotional Eating

Apart from the urge for women to eat more when they work out and the love for sugary foods, women turn to food for emotional consolation. Emotional eaters do not eat because they are hungry; they eat because they want to feel better. By eating salty, fatty, and sugary foods, they tap into the reward center of the brain, which leads to massive weight gain because when women indulge in emotional eating, they go to the extreme.

CHAPTER 2 – THE BASICS OF INTERMITTENT FASTING FOR WOMEN

In recent times, one of the most popular trends on the internet today is weight loss. Extra weight is a problem which many people (both men and women) try to address today with women facing it more than men for many extra reasons. Childbirth alongside other factors responsible for the change in physiognomy of the female body can lead to excessive weight gain. Speaking generally now, the prevalence of obesity in our society has been on the increase due to easy access to fast foods on the internet as well as a lack of physical activities – elevator use, remotes, and hilariously the use of assistants like Siri for practically everything.

With this obesity comes with many health challenges like heart disease, respiratory disorders and many others. So, with the few sentences mentioned here, we have established one fact and that which is that obesity is not good for anyone. Amidst all the information out there on how to successfully lose weight, one stands out; which is **Intermittent Fasting**.

What is Intermittent Fasting?

In simple terms, intermittent fasting is one of the oldest dietary interventions in the world today. This dietary intervention simply means a larger fasting window and a smaller eating window.

On a deeper context, intermittent fasting is an eating pattern that revolves between periods of fasting and eating. This eating and fitness pattern does not dictate the type of food you eat but rather, the time you should eat.

Fasting has been a constant practice over the years of human evolution. Hunters and ancient gatherers at the beginning did not eat every time as they sometimes found it hard to get food. They did not eat often, sort of like the intermittent fasting today, and they were healthy and strong all the time, not facing most of the health challenges common today. In fact, it is more natural to fast than to eat three meals per day.

Why Intermittent Fasting

Intermittent fasting is beneficial to your health, especially for weight loss. If you are capable of eating clean and going to the gym on a regular basis, one challenge you might have is time. At some point, eating clean becomes a problem because some of these clean foods become boring, and we find it difficult to cope with them.

If this is not the case, something unexpected might happen to you, keeping you away from the gym, and then you put on a lot of weight. Adding this weight suddenly demoralizes you, and suddenly you find yourself ditching your initial weight loss plan.

So, what next. You cannot go to the gym anymore because of your job or some other good reason, eating clean has become boring and hard to keep up with, and you feel like the only thing that can happen to you is for you to keep on putting on weight.

This is where intermittent fasting comes in. Intermittent fasting is a great and flexible way to lose weight even with whatever you eat, and you do not even have to exercise as much as you do with other plans. The primary thing you need is a conscious mindset towards Intermittent fasting because there is room for any food you like – some of it at least. Once you are mindful of your intermittent fasting schedule and you eat reasonably well, you would find results coming your way, even without going to the gym.

Differences Between Intermittent Fasting in Men and Women

We all know that some part of the schedules of intermittent fasting for men and women is the same. However, there is a difference in intermittent fasting between men and women because the female body is susceptible to calorie restrictions. Once you make some changes to your calorie intake as a woman, you find that your body goes through some changes that make life pretty tricky at the beginning.

The average woman needs about 2000 calories daily to be healthy, and that same woman needs about 1500 calories to lose one pound of weight weekly. However, many factors determine how women's hormones are affected by intermittent fasting, such as current weight, metabolic health, age, activity levels, and height.

What are calories?

A calorie is an energy measuring unit. The energy content of food is measured using calories. If you have to lose weight, you must eat fewer calories than your body consumes each day. If as a woman, you do not fast properly – fasting too frequent or too long – your hypothalamus is affected, and you find yourself having hormonal imbalances, ones that can even affect your menstrual cycle.

This is the reason for this book, as we look to cover intermittent fasting for women in such a way that it does not affect your hormones in any way. We are going to be covering al lot of ground and using tools such as alternate fasting, fewer fasting days, non-fasting days, and shorter fasting periods.

HEALTH BENEFITS OF INTERMITTENT FASTING FOR WOMEN

The major benefit of intermittent fasting for women is that it helps you lose weight as a woman, particularly your waistline, which is what many women want. However, there are other health benefits associated with taking on intermittent fasting as a woman, including reducing the risk of a number of serious diseases.

Improves Heart health

The leading cause of both men and women's death worldwide is heart disease. Health challenges like high LDL cholesterol, high blood pressure, and high triglyceride concentrations are some of the principal factors for the development of heart disease.

With intermittent fasting for women, one thing is sure, you have you are provided with a means to not only lose weight but a means to lose weight that does not leave you uncomfortable with hormonal challenges in the process.

Once you start the process of Intermittent fasting you definitely reduce caloric intake which is the number one factor that leads to reduced heart health as well as other health challenges that might possibly lead to poor heart health.

Helps Prevent and Cope with Diabetes

For women who feel their lifestyle and eating methods can lead to health challenges like diabetes and for women who already have diabetes who are looking to live a proper life even with the disease, intermittent fasting is your best bet at that. Intermittent fasting does not only reduce the number of calories, it also helps reduce the amount of insulin in the body as well as insulin resistance.

Intermittent fasting for more than 10 weeks has been shown to lower insulin levels by a whopping 25%. It does not stop there; it also helps reduce blood sugar by 5% in women with diabetes.

Helps with Weight loss

Intermittent fasting is one of the simplest and most effective way to lose weight for women, particularly if done effectively. Short term intermittent fasting, is more effective than other forms of calorie restrictions.

Rather than running on energy from the food you just ate, fasting enables your body to take advantage of stores. Fat which amasses in the body is used at whatever point food supply becomes low. This leads to moderate, steady weight loss that can be a genuine advantage.

Since fasting is fused as a way of life rather than an impermanent fix, this sort of diet is substantially more sustainable than numerous other "crash diet plans." Intermittent fasting is a significant, reliable method for weight loss and muscle gain. At first, you'll see a checked weight loss because of losing water weight. Be that as it may, with intermittent fasting, every day you fast will show a weight loss of 0.5 pounds of pure fat.

Improves Glucose Tolerance

For people with diabetes, fasting can be an excellent way to regulate glucose and even enhance glucose tolerance. Anybody searching for a unique way to increase insulin sensitivity should try an intermittent fast. The impacts of fasting can have positive effects on how your body forms glucose.

By and large, insulin sensitivity is the by-product of accumulating glucose in tissues that aren't meant to be stored. As the body consumes stored fat, that excess accumulation winds up smaller and smaller. This permits the cells in your tissues and liver to become increasingly receptive to insulin.

Improves Metabolism

Some of the reason intermittent fasting causes you to get in shape is that the limitation of food, followed by eating times, improves your digestion. While long-term fasting can, in reality, moderate your metabolism, shorter fasts when on intermittent fasting have been demonstrated to increase metabolism. Indeed, as much as up to 15 percent.

This is a more compelling instrument than long-term calorie restrictions, which is not the best for the body's digestion. Weight loss often goes with muscle loss. Furthermore, since muscle tissue consumes calories, reducing muscle mass prompts a drop in your body's capacity to process food. Intermittent fasting keeps your digestion running efficiently by helping you keep up your muscle tissue as much as could reasonably be expected.

Stimulates Brain Function

Intermittent fasting may have "huge implications for mental wellbeing." It stimulates the brain in various ways: improves the development of neurons, helps in recuperation following a stroke or other brain damages, and improves memory performance. Intermittent fasting may help reduce the danger of developing neurodegenerative infections like Parkinson's or Alzheimer's. There's proof to demonstrate that it might, in reality, even improve both personal capacity and personal satisfaction for individuals living with those conditions at the moment.

Helps improve self-confidence

Intermittent fasting is something that has to do with the body and how you feel about yourself. Most individuals who decide to go on the adventure of intermittent fasting have one goal in mind asides other essential factors, and that is to lose weight. Why do you want to lose weight as a woman? It is basically to look better and feel much better about yourself. You remember when you were much younger, mainly before you started putting on weight and you wish that you could go back to the way you were before, particularly women who have given birth. Intermittent fasting helps you lose that weight, which boosts your self-confidence and how you feel about yourself. One of the important things that low self-esteem from excess weight gain can cause is depression and depression has been one of the primary reasons for many deaths today making intermittent fasting and the resulting weight loss a lifesaver and confidence booster.

CHAPTER 3 – TYPES OF INTERMITTENT FASTING FOR WOMEN

There is no single strategy when it comes to dieting. This also applies to the types of intermittent fasting. In general, women should always approach fasting more comfortable than men, I'll tell you why. This may include fewer days of fasting shorter periods of fasting, and/or a small amount of calories on the days of fasting.

Here are some of the best kinds of intermittent fasting for women:

Crescendo Fasting: for two to three days a week, fasting 12–16 hours. Fasting days should be non-consecutive and uniformly spaced throughout the week. An example is Tuesday, Thursday, Saturday. You can see the spacing here.

Eat-stop-eat fasting: this is a plan also known as the 24 hours protocol where a woman fasts for a complete 24-hour once or twice a week. Start with fasts of 14–16 hours and build up slowly.

The 5:2 diet: this fast is also known to some as the fast diet. Here you limit calories for two days a week to 25 percent of your usual intake and eat as you usually do for the other five days. Allow a day between days of fasting to help you get accustomed to this fasting type.

Alternate-Day Fasting – Modified: This involves you fasting every other day but eating on non-fasting days as usual. On a fasting day, you are allowed to consume 25% of your usual calorie intake and on non-fasting days as much as you usually do.

The 16/8 Method: This involves fasting 16 hours a day and eating all the calories you need within an eight-hour window. As we said in the beginning, it is recommended that women begin with 14-hour fasts and eventually create up to 16 hours.

Whatever you choose, eating well during the non-fasting periods is still essential. You may not experience the same weight loss and health benefits if you eat a large amount of unhealthy, calorie-dense foods during the non-fasting periods.

The best strategy at the end of the day is one that you can tolerate and maintain in the long run, and that does not have any adverse health effects. Women can do intermittent fasting in many ways. The 5:2 diet, alternate-day fasting, and crescendo fasting are some of the most excellent techniques.

How to Get Started.

In reality, you have tried many intermittent fasts before. Many individuals eat this way instinctively, skipping meals in the morning or at night. The simplest way to get started is to select and give one of the intermittent techniques of fasting above a try. You do not necessarily need to follow a structured plan, though. Fasting whenever it fits you is an option. It can work for some people to skip meals from time to time when you don't feel hungry or don't have time to cook.

It doesn't matter what kind of fast you choose at the end of the day. Looking for a technique that works best for you and your lifestyle is the most significant thing. Choosing one of the above techniques and giving it a go is the easy way to get began. If you experience any adverse effects, stop instantly.

SIDE EFFECTS AND SAFETY OF INTERMITTENT FASTING

For most women, modified variants of intermittent fasting seem like a safe way to start. That said, several studies have reported some side effects on fasting days, including hunger, mood swings, absence of concentration, decreased energy, headaches, and poor breath. There are also some internet tales of women reporting that their menstrual cycle has stopped after an intermittent fasting diet.

You should consult your doctor before starting intermittent fasting.

If you have medical conditions such as:

- Having a history of eating disorders
- If you have diabetes or experience low levels of blood sugar regularly.

- If you are skinny, malnourished, or have deficiencies in nutrition.
- If you are pregnant, breastfeeding or trying to conceive.
- If you have fertility issues or an amenorrhea history.

Intermittent fasting seems to have a decent safety profile at the end of the day. However, if you encounter any problems, stop immediately.

Hunger, low energy, bad breath, and headaches can be caused by intermittent fasting. Women pregnant, attempting to conceive or having a history of eating disorders should seek medical guidance before beginning an intermittent fasting scheme.

The intermittent fasting of the bottom line is a nutritional pattern involving periodic, short-term fasts. Women's best kinds include regular fasts of 14–16 hours, a 5:2 diet or altered alternate-day fasting.

While intermittent fasting is useful to heart health, diabetes, and weight loss, some proof suggests that some females may have adverse impacts on breeding and blood sugar concentrations. That said, altered variants of intermittent fasting seem secure for most females and maybe a more appropriate choice than more extended or more stringent fasts. If you're a woman who wants to lose weight or enhance her health, it's certainly

How Intermittent Fasting Affects Your Cells and Hormones as a Woman

When you fast, a lot of things happen in your body on the molecular and cellular level.

For example, your body regulates hormone levels to make stored body fat more available for use.

Your cells also change the expression of genes and initiate essential repair processes.

Here are some changes that happen to your body when you go on an intermittent fast:

- **Cellular repair:** When on an intermittent fast, your cells cellular repair processes. This includes autophagy, where cells remove and digest old and dysfunctional proteins that build up in the cells
- **Gene expression:** These are changes in the function of genes related to protection against disease and longevity.
- **Human Growth Hormone:** The levels of growth hormone become very high, increasing as much as five times. This has benefits for muscle gain and fat loss, to name a few.
- **Insulin sensitivity:** levels of insulin drop dramatically, and Insulin sensitivity improves.

Lower insulin levels make stored body fat reachable for use.

These changes in cell function, hormone levels, and gene expression are responsible for the health benefits of intermittent fasting.

Weight loss and muscle gain is the most common reason why people try intermittent fasting making it essential to this book.

By making you eat smaller meals, intermittent fasting can lead to an automatic reduction in calorie intake, giving you a chance not only to lose weight but also to work on your muscles.

Also, intermittent fasting changes hormone levels to help weight loss. In addition to lowering your insulin and increasing growth hormone levels in the body, it increases the release of norepinephrine (the fat-burning hormone).

CAN YOU PRACTICE A QUICK WORKOUT WHILE ON A FAST?

If for other reasons you're trying Intermittent fasting or you're fasting and you still want to get your workouts in, there are some pros and cons to consider before you decide to work out in a fasted state.

Some study demonstrates that exercising while fasting impacts the biochemistry of muscles and metabolism associated with insulin sensitivity and constant blood sugar concentrations control. Research also promotes eating and exercising instantly before digestion or absorption takes place. For anyone with type 2 diabetes or metabolic syndrome, this is particularly crucial.

An upside while fasting is that your stored carbohydrates are most probably depleted, so you're going to burn more fat to fuel your exercise. However, studies on this are small and countered by Trusted Source studies saying that when you work on an empty stomach, you don't burn more fat.

Sounds like a victory the potential to burn more fat? There is a downside before you jump on the fasted cardio trend.

It is feasible that your body will begin breaking down muscle while exercising in a fasted state to use protein for fuel. "Moreover, you're more likely to hit the wall, meaning you're going to have less energy and not be able to work as hard or execute as well."

Are you supposed to fast while you work out?

If you are set to try intermittent fasting while continuing your workout routine, there are some things you can do to make your workout efficient.

1. Think through timing

There are three factors when it comes to making your workout faster: whether you should practice before, during, or after the fueling window. One popular intermittent fasting technique is the 16:8 protocol. The idea relates to consuming all food within an eight-hour fueling window and then a 16-hour fast.

"Working out in front of the window is perfect for someone who works well on an empty stomach during practice, while during the window it is better suited for someone who does not like exercising on an empty stomach and who also intends to capitalize on nutrition after workout.

2. Choose the type of workout based on your macros

It's important to pay attention to the macronutrients you take the day before and after you exercise. "For example, strength workouts usually require more carbohydrates on the day, while cardio / high-intensity training interval can be done on a lower carb day.

3. After your workout, eat the correct meals to construct or retain muscle

The best option to combine intermittent fasting and practice is to schedule your workouts during your eating periods so that your nutritional level is high. "And intermittent fasting you're doing heavy lifting having protein after the exercise is essential for your body to help with regeneration.

In 30 minutes after your exercise, follow up any strength training with carbohydrates and about 20 grams of protein.

HOW CAN YOU PRACTICE FASTING SAFELY?

The achievement of any exercise program or weight loss relies on how secure it is to be sustained over time. You need to remain in the secure area intermittent fasting your ultimate objective is to reduce body fat and keep your fitness level while doing intermittent fasting. Here are some tips from experts to assist you do just that.

- **Eat a meal near your medium-to high-intensity workout**

This is where the timing of meals comes into play. Khorana claims it's essential to timing a dinner close to a workout of moderate or high intensity. This way your body can tap into some glycogen shops to fuel your exercise.

- **Staying hydrated**

It doesn't mean removing water to remember fasting. In reality, while fasting, he advises that you drink more water.

- **Keep up your electrolytes**

A useful source of low-calorie hydration is coconut water. "It replenishes electrolytes, has low calories and a nice taste. Sports drinks are high in sugar, so prevent excessive drinking.

- **Keep the intensity and length relatively low**

Take a break intermittent fasting you push yourself too hard and start feeling dizzy or light-headed. It's essential to listen to your body.

- **Consider the type of fast you want**

If you're doing an intermittent 24-hour fast, you should stick to low-intensity workouts like walking, restorative yoga, or mild pilates. But if you do the quick 16:8, much of the 16-hour fasting window is night, sleep, and early in the day, so it's not as critical to stick to some kind of practice.

- **Listen to your body**

Listening to your body is the most significant advice to listen to when practicing during intermittent fasting. "Intermittent fasting you begin to feel weak or dizzy, you may experience low or dehydrated blood sugar. Intermittent fasting that is the case, she will immediately choose a carbohydrate-electrolyte beverage and then follow up with a well-balanced dinner.

While some individuals may be experiencing exercise and intermittent fasting, others may not feel comfortable doing any type of practice while fasting. Before beginning any nutrition or exercise program, check with your doctor or health care provider.

INTERMITTENT FASTING TIPS FOR BEGINNERS

Intermittent fasting is a very popular health and fitness trend today in which people use to lose weight, simplify their lifestyle and improve their health.

Intermittent fasting is a pattern of eating that cycles between fasting and eating periods. The thing about intermittent fasting is that it is not specifically about what you eat but when you eat. With this in mind, this is not a diet in the conventional sense but somewhat ab eating pattern.

Intermittent fasting is somewhat easy to achieve if you know the right way to go about it and, in this article, we offer you 7 intermittent fasting tips for beginners, let's go.

- **Pick a plan that suits your lifestyle**

Intermittent fasting is something that has to fit the lifestyle of the person who has chosen to make intermittent fasting a part of his life irrespective of the reason why. If you choose a pattern of intermittent fasting just because someone else chose that eating pattern, then there is a high probability of it failing quickly especially if the lifestyle of the person you have chosen to copy does not match yours. Therefore, knowing fully well that there are different types of intermittent fasting, sit down and carefully select the one that would perfectly suit you.

- **Start off slow**

Nobody achieves anything without slow and humble beginnings. Rome was not built in a day and keeping this in mind you would understand that you do not have to rush yourself. intermittent fasting is not a quick fix and rushing a fasting program just because you want to see immediate results is not the way to go. Follow the fast type which you have decided to engage with and slowly engage with persistence as this way, you would achieve your desires for choosing intermittent fasting without any problems whatsoever.

- **Drink a lot of water**

Water is a very great choice all day long everyday more so when on intermittent fasting. You can take still or sparkling water depending on the one you enjoy. The most important thing is that you stay away from any form of artificially sweetened water or enhancers like crystal light because these artificial sweeteners do major damages to your insulin levels, destroying your reason for fasting in the first place.

- **Drink black coffee in the morning**

Black coffee is a beverage that is calorie free and is taken by many people during intermittent fasting without any side effects. Irrespective of what type of coffee (caffeinated and decaffeinated) taking coffee in the morning is fine just not with any sweetener or milk. Black coffee in the morning enhances the benefits of intermittent fasting and a study has shown that an early intake of increases ketone production which means you are likely to burn fat from that time. Coffee especially in the morning improves insulin sensitivity, which means more stable blood sugar.

- **Keep busy while fasting**

Intermittent fasting is better while working because if you do not have time to eat due to the fact that you are always on the move, the fasting time and process for so many reasons would seem and feel easier than it normally would when you would just sit around and wonder when the time for the next meal would finally come. Some of the reasons intermittent fasting is simpler while working are:

- It takes less time
- You're less hungry
- Mental clarity

- **Don't overdo it during the feeding window**

Intermittent fasting as we know somewhat has to do with eating and fasting sequentially where during the eating periods, there are no constrains concerning what is and what is not to be eaten. The point we are trying to bring out is that during the window of eating, overdoing it is not an option as the essence of the intermittent fasting would have been defeated.

- **Follow a low-carb diet between fasting periods**

A low-carb diet is one that assures us for a fact that while eating when on an intermittent fast, we consume little or no fat at all. With the consumption of little or no fat, the body goes into ketosis, a state in which when it is reached assures us of optimum weight loss. This assures us a win as one of the major reasons for intermittent fasting is weight loss.

Intermittent fasting is something that many understand and many others do not. The major question here is, do we understand it enough? In every quest we go through in life either physical or mental, we have to understand that someone else has been there and has scaled through.

Intermittent fasting today is a very broad and well talked about topic today as many have testified of their inability to make the best out of their intermittent fasting tryouts.

With all that we have heard from individuals as problems relating to successful fasting, these tips for beginners would make the adventure of intermittent fasting a lot easier than it would have been.

CHAPTER 4 – TYPES OF WEIGHT LOSS DIET PLANS

There are a lot of diets for weight loss out there. Some focus on reducing your hunger, while others limit calories, carbs, or fat. Since every one of them guarantees to be superior, it very well may be challenging to know which one's merit attempting.

In this section of the e-book, we look at some of the standard weight loss diet plans and the science behind them.

THE PALEO DIET

The paleo diet claims that you ought to eat similar foods that your ancestors ate before the development of agriculture.

The hypothesis is that most current illnesses can be connected to Western diets and the utilization of grains, processed foods, and dairy.

While it's doubtful whether this diet indeed gives similar nourishments your ancestors ate, it is connected to a few fantastic medical advantages.

How it works: The paleo diet stresses whole foods, lean protein, vegetables, natural products, nuts, and seeds, while discouraging processed foods, sugar, grains, and dairy.

Some increasingly flexible versions of the paleo diet likewise take into consideration dairy like cheese and margarine, just as tubers like sweet potatoes and potatoes.

Weight loss: Several examinations have demonstrated that the paleo diet can prompt colossal weight loss and reduced waist measure.

Other benefits: The diet appears to be successful at diminishing danger factors for heart illness, for example, blood triglycerides, cholesterol, glucose, and circulatory strain.

The drawback: The paleo diet eliminates vegetables, whole grains, and dairy, which are stable and nutritious.

THE VEGAN DIET

The veggie lover diet confines every animal product for ecological, or wellbeing reasons.

How it Works: Veganism is the strictest type of vegetarianism.

Notwithstanding taking out meat, it also eliminates dairy, eggs, and animal-derived items, for example, egg whites, whey, gelatin, nectar, casein, and a few types of vitamin D3.

Weight loss: A vegan diet is by all accounts extremely compelling at helping individuals shed pounds — regularly without checking calories — because its low fat and high fiber content may make you feel full for longer.

Vegetarian diets are reliably connected to bring down bodyweight, and body mass index (BMI) contrasted with different diet plans.

Nonetheless, calorie for calorie, vegetarian diets are not more viable for weight loss than other different diets.

Weight loss on vegan diets is necessarily connected with decreased calorie consumption.

Other benefits: Plant-based diets are connected to a decreased danger of type 2 diabetes, coronary illness, and premature death.

Constraining processed meat may likewise decrease your danger of Alzheimer's sickness and death from coronary illness or cancer.

The drawback: Because vegetarian diets eliminate animal foods, they might be low in a few nutrients, including iron, calcium, zinc, vitamin B12, vitamin D, iodine, and omega-3 unsaturated fat.

THE KETO DIET

Keto diets have been popular for a considerable length of time — particularly for weight loss.

There are a few kinds of keto diets. However, all include restricting carb intake to 20– 150 grams every day.

The essential point of the eating plan is to compel your body to use more fats for fuel as opposed to utilizing carbs as a fundamental wellspring of energy.

How it works: Keto diets underline unlimited measures of protein and fat while extremely restricting your carb consumption.

At the point when carb consumption is exceptionally low, unsaturated fats are transported into your blood and then transported to your liver, where some of them are transformed into ketones.

Your body would then be able to use unsaturated fats and ketones without carbs as its essential energy source.

Weight loss: Numerous investigations show that the keto diet is amazingly useful for weight loss, particularly in overweight and fat people.

They appear to be viable at decreasing hazardous belly fat, which can lodge around your organs.

Individuals on very keto diets generally achieve a state called ketosis. Numerous examinations take note of that ketogenic diet leads to more than double the weight loss than a low-fat, calorie-limited diet.

Other benefits: Keto diets will, in general decrease your cravings and make you feel less hungry, prompting an automatic reduction in calorie consumption.

Besides, keto diets may benefit many significant illness risk factors, for example, blood triglycerides, glucose levels, insulin levels, cholesterol levels, and blood pressure.

The drawback: Keto diet sometimes fall short for everybody. Some feel good on them while others feel hopeless.

A few people may encounter an expansion in "bad" LDL cholesterol.

In incredibly exceptional cases, very keto diets can cause a severe condition called ketoacidosis. This condition is by all accounts progressively basic in lactating ladies and can be severe whenever left untreated. In any case, keto diets are alright for most individuals.

THE DUKAN DIET

The Dukan diet is a low-carb high-protein weight loss diet split into four stages — two weight loss stages and two maintenance stages.

To what extent you remain in each stage relies upon how much weight you have to lose. Each step has a dietary pattern.

How it works: The weight loss stages are primarily based on eating healthy high-protein nourishments and compulsory oat grain.

Alternate stages include including non-starchy vegetables pursued by some carbs and fat. Later on, there will be less and less pure protein days to keep up your new weight.

Weight loss: Numerous different investigations demonstrate that high-protein, keto diets may have real weight reduction benefits. These include a higher metabolic rate, a reduction in the hunger hormone ghrelin, and an expansion in a few fullness hormones.

Other benefits: Apart from weight reduction, there are no recorded advantages of the Dukan diet in logical writing.

The drawback: There is next to no quality research accessible on the Dukan diet.

The Dukan diet reduces both fat and carbs — a procedure not founded on science. Expending fat as a significant aspect of a high-protein diet appears to increment metabolic rate contrasted with both low-carb and low-fat eating regimens.

Additionally, quick weight loss accomplished by extreme calorie limitation will, in general reason cause significant muscle loss.

The loss of muscle and severe calorie limitation may likewise make your body preserve energy, making it simple to recover the weight in the wake of losing it.

THE ULTRA-LOW-FAT DIET

An ultra-low-fat diet limits your utilization of fat to under 11% of daily calories.

By and large, a low-fat diet gives around 30% of its calories as fat. Studies show that this diet plan is inadequate for weight loss in the long haul.

Enthusiasts of the ultra-low-fat diet claim that typical low-fat diets are not low enough in fat and that fat admission needs to remain under 10% of total calories to deliver medical advantages and weight loss.

How it works: A ultra-low-fat diet contains 10% or fewer calories from fat. The diet is, for the most part, plant-based and has a constrained admission of animal items.

In this manner, it's commonly extremely high in carbs — around 81% of calories — and low in protein — at 11% of calories.

Weight loss: This diet has demonstrated to be useful for weight loss among fat people.

Other benefits: Studies show that ultra-low-fat diets can increase a few hazard factors for coronary illness, including hypertension, elevated cholesterol, and markers of inflammation.

Shockingly, this high-carb, low-fat diet can likewise prompt critical improvements in type II diabetes.

Besides, it might moderate the movement of multiple sclerosis — an immune system ailment that influences optic nerves in the eyes, your mind, and spinal cord.

The drawback: The fat confinement may cause long term issues, as fat assumes numerous vital jobs in your body. These include helping build cell hormones and membranes, just as helping your body retain fat-soluble vitamins.

Also, an ultra-low-fat diet cuts off the intake of numerous sound nourishments need assortment and is incredibly challenging to stick to.

THE ATKINS DIET

The Atkins diet is the most outstanding low-carb weight loss diet.

Its followers demand that you can get in shape by eating as much protein and fat as you like, as long as you dodge carbs.

The principle motivation behind why keto diets are so viable for weight loss is that they decrease your craving. This makes you eat fewer calories without contemplating it.

How it works: The Atkins diet is part into four stages. It begins with an induction stage, amid which you eat under 20 grams of carbs every day for about fourteen days.

Alternate stages include gradually reintroducing sound carbs once again into your diet as you approach your objective weight.

Weight loss: when it comes to weight loss, the Atkins diet has been studied broadly and found to prompt quicker weight loss than low-fat diets.

Different examinations take note that keto diets are beneficial for weight loss. They are particularly useful in reducing tummy fat, the most dangerous fat that lodges itself in your abdominal cavity.

Other benefits: Numerous examinations demonstrate that keto diet, similar to the Atkins diet, may reduce many risk factors for sickness, including blood triglycerides, cholesterol, glucose, insulin, and pulse.

Compared with other weight-loss diets, keto diets likewise better enhance glucose, "great" HDL cholesterol, triglycerides, and other health markers.

The drawback: As do other keto diets, and the Atkins diet is safe and sound for the vast majority yet may cause issues in rare cases.

THE HCG DIET

The HCG diet is an excellent diet intended to cause rapid weight loss of up to 1–3 pounds every day.

Its users guarantee that it supports digestion and fat misfortune without prompting hunger.

HCG is a hormone present at high levels during early pregnancy.

It tells a lady's body it's pregnant and keeps up the production of hormones that are imperative for fetal improvement. It has additionally been utilized to treat fertility issues.

How it works: The diet is part into three stages. Amid the main stage, you start taking HCG supplements.

Amid the second stage, you pursue an ultra-low-calorie diet of just 550 calories for each day, alongside HCG supplement drops, pellets, infusions, or sprays. The weight-loss stage is recommended for 3–6 weeks at any given moment.

In the third stage, you quit taking HCG and gradually increase your food consumption.

Weight loss: The HCG diet causes weight loss, yet different investigations presume that the weight loss is because of the ultra-low-calorie diet alone — not the HCG hormone.

Moreover, HCG was not found to reduce hunger.

Other benefits: Aside from weight reduction, there are no recorded advantages of the HCG diet.

The drawback: Like most other ultra-low-calorie diets, the HCG diet may cause muscle loss, which results in a decreased capacity to consume calories.

Such extreme calorie confinement further diminishes the number of calories your body consumes. This is because your body believes it's starving and along these lines endeavors to preserve energy.

Also, most HCG products available are tricks and don't contain any HCG. Just injections can raise blood levels of this hormone.

Besides, the eating diet has many symptoms, headaches, weariness, and depression. There is likewise one report of a lady developing blood pressure, probably brought about by the diet.

The FDA objects to this diet, marking it unsafe, illicit, and fake.

THE ZONE DIET

The Zone Diet is a low-glycemic diet that makes you limit carbs to 32– 45% of daily calories, protein, and fat to 30% each.

It recommends eating just carbs with a low glycemic list (GI).

The GI of a food is a gauge of the amount it raises your blood glucose levels after consumption.

The Zone Diet was at first created to lessen diet-initiated inflammation, cause weight loss, and decrease your danger of perpetual diseases.

How it works: The Zone Diet suggests offsetting every meal with 2/3 fruits, 1/3 protein, and a dash of fat — specifically monounsaturated oil, for example, avocado, olive oil, or almonds.

It likewise limits high-GI carbs, for example, rice, bananas, and potatoes.

Weight loss: Studies on low-GI eating diets are relatively conflicting. While some state that the diet increases weight loss and decreases craving, others show next to no weight loss contrasted with different eating plans.

Other benefits: The best advantage of this diet is a decrease in risk factors for heart illness, for example, reduced cholesterol and triglycerides.

One examination recommends that the Zone Diet may improve glucose control and lower chronic inflammation in overweight or obese people with type II diabetes.

The drawback: One of a couple of downsides of this eating regimen is that it restricts the utilization of some solid carb sources, for example, bananas and potatoes.

With all these diet plans, we look to further buttress on the keto diet, which is a significant part of where we are going in this book.

WHAT IS THE KETO DIET?

The keto diet is a low carb high fat diet which has many benefits. Following this diet is a tool for weight loss and according to studies, this type of diet reduces the risk of certain diseases like epilepsy, heart diseases, stroke, diabetes, Alzheimer's, and many more.

On the keto diet, the body enters a metabolic state known as ketosis. When the body goes into ketosis, it uses ketone bodies as a source of energy instead of the usual source, which was formerly glucose.

Ketone bodies are energy sources derived from fat which are more stable as a source of energy compared to glucose which is primarily derived from carbohydrates.

This metabolic state which is known as ketosis, take anywhere from four days to a week to enter. The minute you enter into ketosis, your body would be using fat as a source of instead of carbs, and this includes not only the fat you eat but the fat stored in the body as well.

With this in mind, when we switch to a ketogenic diet, we change the energy supply of the body to run primarily on fat, burning most of the body fat throughout the day. With the reduction of carbs consumed, the body goes short of that source until It becomes depleted, burning fat more rapidly as a source of energy. Burning fat is not the only advantage of being in the ketogenic diet as we also experience less hunger with steady energy supply.

Benefits of The Ketogenic Diet

Various advantages accompany being on keto from weight reduction and increased health levels to restorative therapeutic applications. Anybody can profit by eating a low-carb, high-fat diet as far as it's done correctly. In this section, you'll find a short and informative rundown of the advantages you can get from a ketogenic diet. Let's go.

1. Controlled Blood Sugar

Keto usually brings glucose levels due to the kind of nourishment you eat. Numerous studies even demonstrate that the ketogenic diet is a more viable approach to oversee and forestall diabetes contrasted with other diets.

In case you have Type II diabetes, you ought to honestly consider a ketogenic diet as it solves many problems associated with the disease. We have numerous testimonies on the subject matter that have had massive success with their glucose control on keto without any issues whatsoever.

2. Mental Focus

Various individuals use the ketogenic diet, particularly for the increased mental performance it brings into the picture.

Ketones are an enormous reservoir of energy for the human brain. When you bring down carb consumption, you keep away from massive spikes in glucose. Together, this can result in improved concentration and fixation (concentration and focus).

Studies demonstrate that an increase in intake of unsaturated fats can have decisive advantages to our brain's capacity.

3. Normalized Hunger and Increased energy

By giving your body a more dependable and superior energy source, you will feel more empowered throughout the day. Fats are seen to be the best molecule to consume as fuel.

Over that, fat usually is all the more fulfilling and winds up, dropping us in a peaceful state for a longer duration of time.

4. Epilepsy

One of the fundamental advantages of the ketogenic diet and epilepsy is that it enables fewer prescriptions to be utilized while as yet offering brilliant control.

Over the most recent couple of years, studies have additionally indicated tremendous results as well in grown-ups treated with keto too.

5. Insulin Resistance

Insulin resistance can prompt type II diabetes whenever left unmanaged. A high measure of research demonstrates that a low carb, the ketogenic diet can help individuals to bring down their levels of insulin to solid extents.

Regardless of whether you're athletic or not, you can profit by insulin reduction on keto through eating nourishments high in omega-3 unsaturated fats.

6. Skin inflammation/acne

It's normal to encounter changes in your skin when you change to a ketogenic diet.

Research demonstrates a plausible association between high-carb eating and increased skin inflammation, so it's presumable that keto can help.

For skin break out, it might be helpful to diminish dairy intake and take after a strict skin cleaning routine.

7. Cholesterol and Blood Pressure

A keto diet has appeared to enhance triglyceride levels and cholesterol levels most connected with arterial buildup. All the more particularly low-carb, high-fat diet plans demonstrate a sensational increment in HDL and diminishing in LDL molecule fixation contrasted with low-fat diets.

Numerous investigations on low-carb diets likewise demonstrate better changes in circulatory strains like blood pressure over other dietary methods.

Some pulse/blood pressure issues are related to the abundance of weight, which is a reward since keto tends to prompt weight reduction.

8. Weight loss

This is the most popular and most sought for the mentioned benefits today. The ketogenic diet utilizes your muscle to fat ratio as a vitality source, so there are apparent weight reduction benefits. On keto, your insulin levels drop incredibly, which transforms your body into a fat consuming machine.

Logically, the ketogenic diet has demonstrated better outcomes contrasted with low-fat and high-carb diets; even in the long haul.

As far as this section is concerned, the majority of the benefits have been covered as well as a necessary explanation of the keto diet as well as ketosis.

HOW TO USE INTERMITTENT FASTING ON THE KETO DIET

As we discussed earlier, there are a few intermittent fasting strategies you can attempt, with no approach being correct or off-base. The standard guideline for anybody practicing intermittent fasting is to fast for at least 12 hours, and no longer than 48 hours on end.

The ideal approach to tell which fasting window works for you, and how frequently to fast, is to focus on how you feel. Observe your energy levels, hunger levels, mental capacity, and rest quality.

On the off chance that you find that you're starving for the day, or can hardly endure an exercise when you're fasting, you may need to reduce your fasting window, at that point progressively increase it by one hour every week.

On the other hand, you could reduce your fasting days. It's likewise imperative to ensure that you are consuming enough calories amid your feeding window.

To put it plainly, you can incorporate intermittent fasting on a keto diet, much the same as you could on some other diet plan, (for example, the Dukan diet) — similar guidelines apply. Nonetheless, the key advantage to intermittent fasting on the keto diet is that it might help kickstart ketosis and help you achieve your health and fitness objectives sooner.

Here are a couple of test calendars to kick you off:

• Eat from 9 am-9 pm, at that point fast for 12 hours.

- Eat from 9 am-7 pm, at that point fast for 14 hours.
- Eat from 12-8 pm, at that point fast for 16 hours.

BENEFITS OF INTERMITTENT FASTING ON THE KETO DIET

1. Entering Ketosis Sooner

Since the keto diet is intended to drive the body into running on ketones from an extremely low carb consumption, you are already fasting of carbs and glucose. This imitates the real fasting that happens with intermittent fasting."

As it were, since you're as of now restricting your body's essential fuel source on the keto diet, including a fasting window can kickstart your body into ketosis sooner. To sweeten the deal, you may think that it's less demanding to fast for longer timeframes since you've just had a short introduction to fasting on the keto diet. A few sources propose intermittent fasting on the keto diet may help dispose of the side effects of keto influenza.

2. Quickening Weight Loss

The keto diet works for breaking weight loss levels in various ways. In the first place, it causes you to consume fat for energy rather than carbs, which controls your digestion to consume put away fat faster. A high-fat diet additionally is all the more satisfying because fats take more time to process than some other nutrients. This forestalls unnecessary eating and additional caloric intake for the day.

Combining the keto diet with intermittent fasting makes a considerably smaller eating window, which enables your body to utilize the food you're eating just as fuel, without feeling hungry.

3. Balancing Blood Sugar

Both the keto diet and intermittent fasting have been shown to enhance insulin sensitivity and balance glucose levels, which is essential for weight reduction — particularly around the midsection. Since the two diet plans can stabilize glucose levels, adopting a combined strategy might be useful for those with type 2 diabetes.

Stable glucose levels likewise help kill mind haze, just as enhance concentration, focus, and memory.

4. Improving Nutrient Absorption

One investigation demonstrated that carb and protein ingestion was increasingly proficient in the individuals who did fasted cardio before eating a meal, contrasted, and the individuals who had a carb-rich breakfast before working out. This proposes fasting can enable your body to utilize nutrients from your post-exercise meals all the more productively, which may quicken the development of lean muscle mass.

5. Promoting Natural Detoxification

Both intermittent fasting and the keto diet trigger a natural procedure in the body called autophagy. Autophagy signifies "self-eating." While this may sound startling at first, autophagy is like your body's internal housekeeping framework to remove, detoxify, and reconstruct healthier cells.

Autophagy usually happens amid times of fasting, or when your protein and carb admission is low. Combining the two techniques can help quicken this procedure, which may decrease your hazard for cardiovascular diseases and type 2 diabetes.

Who Shouldn't Practice Intermittent Fasting on A Keto Diet?

Combining intermittent fasting and the keto diet may not be a solid match for everybody. We suggest you don't practice intermittent fasting if you are:

- Nursing mother

- Pregnant

- Under constant stress

- Struggle with sleep issues, or experience difficulty sleeping

- Have a background marked by eating disorders, for example, bulimia or anorexia

While combining intermittent fasting with the keto diet can enable you to accomplish your health and fitness objectives faster, it's vital to remember that the two diet plans are intended to be used as a part of a sound way of life. Scarcely any things can replace a diet wealthy in whole, nutrient-dense foods.

In case you're merely beginning on the keto diet, it's a smart thought to give your body no less than 3 to 4 weeks to adjust before adding times of intermittent fasting to the blend.

THE REASON WHY OUR KETO DIET DIFFERS FROM OTHER KETO DIETS

In this e-book, we tend to look at the keto diet from another perspective as we look to shine light on better ways to help us attain our weight loss and muscle gain objectives.

Now we know that the typical keto diet consists of about 15-20% protein, leaving fat at a whopping 75% high and carbs between 5-10%.

We also know that weight loss and muscle gain, primarily essentially need protein for success. Making fat the primary source of energy for the body basically would not cut it, especially for individuals who want to lose weight and gain muscle mass.

In the light of this, our keto diet consists of 45% protein (making this the principal component), 35% fat, making it possible to induce ketosis and 20% carbs making exercising less of a drag.

This keto diet, combined with intermittent fasting, as highlighted earlier, can yield marvelous results for weight loss and muscle building, rapidly producing results.

The next section shows our special 3-week diet plan based on our keto diet percentage as well as shopping lists to make this new keto adventure one to be much remembered.

	Breakfast	Lunch	Dinner	Total Macros
Sunday	Breakfast burrito with beans	Sesame Pork Lettuce Wraps.	Mediterranean tuna panini	Calories: 1,520 Protein: 120g Fat: 100g Net Carbs: 16g
Monday	Leftover Chorizo Breakfast Bake with 3 Slices	Thick-Cut Bacon	Spiced Pumpkin Soup	Calories: 1,570 Protein: 172g Fat: 104g Net Carbs: 16g
Tuesday	Fruity oatmeal	Easy Beef Curry	Fast-cooked chicken creole	Calories: 1,700 Protein: 163g Fat: 108.5g Net Carbs: 22g

Wednesday	Lemon Poppy Ricotta Pancakes with 3 Slices Thick-Cut Bacon	Rainbow Turkey Kebab	Leftover Rosemary Roasted Chicken and Veggies	Calories: 1,665 Protein: 130g Fat: 95.5g Net Carbs: 23.5g
Thursday	Leftover Lemon Poppy Ricotta Pancakes with 3 Slices Thick-Cut Bacon	Leftover Spiced Pumpkin Soup	Egg salad sandwich with watercress	Calories: 1,540 Protein: 130.5g Fat: 100g Net Carbs: 22.5g
Friday	Sweet Blueberry Coconut Porridge with 1 Slice Thick-Cut Bacon	Leftover Easy Beef Curry	Turkey wraps	Calories: 1,670 Protein: 130g Fat: 94g Net Carbs: 33.5g
Saturday	Blueberry	Leftover Easy	Quinoa, coconut	Calories:

| | mug muffin | Beef Curry | and salted peanut butter cookie dough | 1,625 Protein: 140.5g Fat: 92g Net Carbs: 27g |

14- DAYS KETO DIET MEAL PLAN AND RECIPES ON INTERMITTENT FASTING

WEEK 1

SHOPPING LIST

PROTEIN

- Bacon, thick-cut - 17 slices
- Beef chuck – 1 pound
- Chicken thighs, deboned - 4
- Chorizo sausage – 4 ounces
- Lamb chops, bone-in – 2 (about 6 ounces meat)
- Pork, ground – 6 ounces
- Sausage, Italian – 6 ounces
- Eggs – 7 large ones

DAIRY

- Almond milk, unsweetened – 1 cup
- Butter - 1 pound
- Cheddar cheese, shredded – 2 tablespoons
- Heavy cream – 5 tablespoons
- Mozzarella cheese, shredded– ½ cup
- Ricotta cheese, whole-milk – 6 ounces

PRODUCE

- Asparagus – ¼ pound
- Avocado – 2 medium ones
- Celery – 1 stalk
- Cilantro – 1 bunch
- Lemon – 1 large
- Bell pepper, green – small
- Garlic – 1 head
- Ginger – 1 piece
- Carrots – 2 small ones
- Lime – 1
- Bell pepper, red – 1 medium
- Blueberries – 60g
- Butter lettuce – 4 leaves
- Rosemary – 1 bunch
- Onion, yellow – 2 small, 2 medium ones
- Parsnip – 1 small
- Zucchini – 1 small
- Mushrooms, sliced – 4 ounces

PANTRY ITEMS

- Ground cinnamon
- Ground flaxseed – ¼ cup
- Liquid stevia
- Marinara sauce – ¼ cup
- Olive oil
- Onion powder
- Garlic powder
- Coconut flour – ¼ cup
- Coconut milk, canned – 1 can
- Coconut oil
- Curry powder
- Dried oregano
- Dried thyme
- Egg white protein powder
- Soy sauce
- Powdered erythritol
- Pumpkin puree – ½ cup
- Salt
- Sesame oil
- Poppy seeds – 1 tablespoon
- Almond flour – ¼ cup
- Sesame seeds – 1 tablespoon
- Shaved coconut – ¼ cup
- Pepper
- Ground nutmeg
- Baking powder
- Balsamic vinegar
- Chicken broth – 1 cup

WEEK 1 RECIPES

MEDITERRANEAN TUNA PANINI

Protein: 34 grams

Key benefits: It is wealthy in Omega-3 unsaturated fats from the tuna, in addition to low in calories, cholesterol and saturated fat.

Preparation:

- This is a Mediterranean blend of protein, vegetables and tart taste of lemon juice. Combine light tuna, tomatoes, feta cheddar, artichokes, onion, olives, trick, a teaspoon of lemon squeeze, and ground pepper.
- Spread the tuna blend among 4 cuts of whole wheat bread. Cook the Panini utilizing canola oil over medium heat for two minutes or until one side is golden dark coloured. At that point cook the opposite side for an additional two minutes at that point serve.

FRUITY OATS

Protein: 24 grams

Key benefits: No cooking required, incredible wellspring of fibre, easy to do and you can put any organic products you need.

Preparation:

- This is a standout amongst the most fundamental yet control stuffed breakfast dinners you can do. Cook some dry cereal and blend it with skim milk rather than water.
- Include a few apples and walnuts (since it can enable you to feel full more) or you can blend in your own selection of fruits.
- Remember to sprinkle it with cinnamon and nectar for sweet taste.

RAINBOW TURKEY KEBAB

Protein: 28 grams

Key benefits: A fair carb-protein-vegetable meal that will without a doubt leave your belly happy.

Preparation:

- Cut turkey breast, red, yellow and green peppers into 1-inch squares. Then again stick in the peppers and turkey breast into metal sticks.
- In a little bowl, join half measure of apricot jam, soy sauce, vinegar, salt and pepper.
- Brush this blend over the kebab and marinate it for 30 minutes (or as long as 6 hours in the event that you favour it longer).
- Place the kebabs on medium-high warmth barbecue until turkey is never again pink. You can attempt chicken breast as well.

EGG PLATE OF MIXED GREENS SANDWICH WITH WATERCRESS

Protein: 16 grams

Key benefits: A fast evening fix in addition to the vegetable watercress is rich in phytonutrients and an ideal method to support your evening.

Preparation:

- This recipe is stuffed with protein and less fat and calories. To do this, remove the egg yolks from the hard-boiled eggs and include sour cream, mayonnaise and mustard.
- Cleave the egg whites and include it in the yolk blend at that point season it with salt and pepper.
- Cut in some bread (whole wheat), it would be ideal if you arrange the watercress and spread the egg plate of salad. On the off chance that you don't have watercress, cucumber and lettuce will do.

TURKEY WRAPS

Protein: 27 grams

Key benefits: No cook bite that is fast, simple and exceptionally easy to do. Also, it is both wealthy in protein and fibre content.

Preparation:

- All you need is turkey breast and green lettuce and you are a great idea to go. To do this, simply wrap the turkey breast in green lettuce leaves.
- You can even include cheese in it in spite of the fact that it might include a couple of grams of protein.
- You can likewise roll the turkey with reduced fat Swiss cheese. Simply make a point to go for the whole cut turkey rather than the prepared store meat for lesser sodium content and food additives.

BLUEBERRY MUG MUFFIN

Protein: 8 to 10 grams for every muffin

Key benefits: Lesser calories, fat, sugar and sodium than muffins purchased in pastry kitchens.

Preparation:

- Blend some oats, ¼ crisp or frozen blueberries, a teaspoon of baking powder and olive oil, 2 tablespoon of ground flax, 2 teaspoons cinnamon, 2 egg whites and sugar.
- Blend it all in a microwave-safe compartment and cook it in the microwave for 50 seconds to a minute. Fulfilling your hunger anytime of the day has never been this simple.

QUINOA, COCONUT AND SALTED NUTTY SPREAD TREAT BATTER

Protein: 12 grams

Key benefits: An ideal veggie lover, all natural low-sugar treat to fulfill your sweet tooth.

Preparation:

- Blend ¼ glass regular nutty spread, maple syrup, low-fat coconut cream and extra virgin coconut oil.
- Include sea salt drops and coconut chips.
- At that point include coconut flour, quinoa drops and hacked chocolate.
- Combine everything until it forms into a mixture. This can be served either in its dough form or prepared treats.

BREAKFAST BURRITO WITH BEANS

Protein: 25 grams

Key benefits: Short planning time, easy to make and an extraordinary wellspring of protein.

Preparation:

- This morning meal burrito can be considered as a power breakfast since it has all that you need in a solitary feast.
- All you need is a corn tortilla, fried eggs, onions, dark beans jalapeño, lime juice, cilantro, tomatoes and you're ready.

QUICK COOKED CHICKEN CREOLE

Protein: 33.3 grams

Key benefits: Quick and simple to do, no additional fat and lesser salt substance.

Preparation:

- Cook chicken breast cut into strips until never again pink.
- Include a container of tomatoes (low sodium is ideal), some low sodium bean stew sauce, 1 some green pepper, celery, onion, garlic, a tablespoon of basil and parsley, ¼ teaspoon of smashed pepper, and salt and heat to the point of boiling.
- Give it a chance to stew and cover for 10 minutes. You can serve this over rice or whole wheat pasta.

WEEK 2

	Breakfast	Lunch	Dinner	Total Macros
Sunday	Banana oat protein smoothie	Easy Cheeseburger Salad	Chicken Zoodle Alfredo	Calories: 1,530 Fat: 113.5g Protein: 107.5g Net Carbs: 18.5g
Monday	Cheesy scrambled eggs	Pan-Fried Pepperoni Pizzas	Cabbage and Sausage Skillet	Calories: 1,670 Fat: 129g Protein: 103g Net Carbs: 20.5g
Tuesday	Mozzarella Veggie-Loaded Quiche with 1 Slice Thick-	Leftover Easy Cheeseburger Salad	Fresh Mexican tuna salad	Calories: 1,580 Protein: 117.5g Fat: 104.5g Net

				Cut Bacon			Carbs: 33g
Wednesday	Pepper Jack Sausage Egg Muffins with 3 Slices Thick-Cut Bacon	Crostini with spinach, poached egg and creamy mustard sauce	Leftover Cabbage and Sausage Skillet	Calories: 1,650 Protein: 127g Fat: 101g Net Carbs: 29g
Thursday	Leftover Savory Ham and Cheese Waffles with 1 Slice Thick-Cut Bacon	Leftover Cabbage and Sausage Skillet	Chicken soup for vegetable lovers	Calories: 1,620 Protein: 149g Fat: 88g Net Carbs: 18.5g
Friday	Leftover Pepper Jack Sausage Egg Muffins with 1 Slice Thick-Cut Bacon	Curried chicken pitas	Leftover Gyro Salad with Avo-Tzatziki	Calories: 1,595 Protein: 140g Fat: 95g Net Carbs: 15.5g

| Saturday | Bacon and jalapeno egg sandwich | Leftover Cabbage and Sausage Skillet with 1 Slice Thick-Cut Bacon | Leftover Gyro Salad with Avo-Tzatziki | Calories: 1,605 Protein: 142g Fat: 100g Net Carbs: 22.5g |

SHOPPING LIST

PROTEIN

- Bacon, thick-cut - 11 slices
- Lamb, ground – 1 pound
- Pepperoni, diced – 1 ½ ounces
- Sausage links, Italian – 6 large
- Beef, ground – 7 ounces
- Breakfast sausage – 10 ounces
- Chicken breast – 2 (6-ounce) breasts
- Eggs – 15 large
- Ham, diced – 1 ounce

DAIRY

- Butter – ¾ cup
- Mayonnaise – ½ cup
- Mozzarella cheese, shredded 1 ½ cups
- Cheddar cheese, shredded – ½ cup
- Heavy cream – 1 cup
- Sour cream – ¼ cup
- Whipped cream – ¼ cup
- Parmesan cheese – ¾ cup
- Almond milk, vanilla – ¼ cup
- Pepper jack cheese, shredded – ½ cup

PRODUCE

- Cucumber, English – 1
- Dill – 1 bunch
- Cabbage, green – ½ head
- Lemon – 1
- Avocado – 2 medium
- Basil – 1 bunch
- Chives – 1 bunch
- Tomatoes, cherry – 4
- Mint – 1 bunch
- Romaine lettuce – 7 ½ cups
- Spinach, frozen – ¼ cup
- Tomatoes, diced – 1/3 cup
- Zucchini – 2 cups
- Onion, yellow – 1 medium

PANTRY ITEMS

-
- Dried thyme
- Egg white protein powder, vanilla – 3 scoops (60g)
- Garlic powder
- Powdered erythritol
- Psyllium husk powder
- Almond flour – 6 tablespoons
- Baking powder
- Chicken broth – ¼ cup
- Coconut oil
- Dried oregano
- Salt
- Tomato sauce, low-carb
- Vanilla extract

- Italian seasoning
- Ketchup
- Mustard
- Olive oil
- Paprika, smoked
- Pepper, black
- Pickles

WEEK 2 RECIPES

CHEESY SCRAMBLED EGGS

Protein: 16 grams

Key benefits: This is a simple and protein-stuffed recipe that will leave your stomach fulfilled.

Preparation:

- You should simply to soften unsalted butter over medium warmth, include onions and jalapeno and cook it until soft, at that point blend in eggs, salt and pepper.
- When the eggs are cooked, blend goat cheese and chives and serve it with whole grain toast or English muffin.
- You can likewise utilize other cheese – simply ensure it is natural for lower salt content and not the procedure purified ones.

BACON AND JALAPENO EGG SANDWICH

Protein: 21 grams

Key benefits: This is a nutritious method to begin your morning, because of the protein and starch substance in addition to fiber. Jalapeno is likewise a key factor since it can give your digestion a lift.

Preparation:

- Cook bacon until crisp. At that point put aside.
- Put a whole grain muffin split into half, with the chop side down, in skillet to toast.
- Put aside. Cook a large natural egg and sprinkle it with pepper and cheese.
- At that point move the egg into the biscuit, top it with bacon, jalapeno, cilantro, onion and tomato and you are good to go.

CROSTINI WITH SPINACH, POACHED EGG AND RICH MUSTARD SAUCE

Protein: 13 grams

Key benefits: This protein powerhouse recipe is a decent mix of fats, protein and starches at lesser calories and cholesterol levels. In the meantime, it is a decent wellspring of fiber as well.

Preparation:

- To do this, combine reduced fat sour cream, Dijon mustard, new lemon juice, fresh chives, salt and pepper in a little bowl with water.
- At that point top each cut of toasted whole grain bread with spinach.
- In a pot, boil 2 inches of water at that point include vinegar.
- Split eggs into a glass and delicately slip into water and let it boil for 2-3 minutes. At that point place the poached egg over the spinach and pour the sour cream blend over the egg before serving this meal.

BANANA OAT PROTEIN SMOOTHIE

Protein: 28 grams

Key benefits: This smoothie is wealthy in potassium that protects your heart. It can likewise prevent muscle issues and sustain your blood glucose particularly after a strenuous exercise.

Preparation:

- Mix oats, some plain low-fat yogurt, banana, fat-free milk, 2 teaspoons honey, ground cinnamon and ice until smooth.
- Top it with walnuts or use maple syrup rather than the usual honey for variety.

CURRIED CHICKEN PITAS

Protein: 27 grams

Key benefits: Short preparation time and the recipe is wealthy in magnesium. It is likewise low in saturated fat, sodium, calories and cholesterol.

Preparation:

- Combine 6 tablespoons of non-fat yogurt, ¼ container low-fat mayonnaise, and a tablespoon of curry powder.
- Include cubed chicken breast, diced pear, celery, cranberries and almonds until all is well combined.
- Spread the chicken blend and sprouts in whole wheat pita bread at that point cut it in half.

CHICKEN SOUP FOR VEGETABLE LOVERS

Protein: 31 grams

Key benefits: This vegetable-stuffed recipe is low in carbs, cholesterol and calorie content and in the meantime, wealthy in potassium.

Preparation:

- Warm a tablespoon of extra virgin olive oil over medium-warmth and include chicken chucks.
- When it is fried, remove the chicken and place on a plate.
- At that point cook the dices zucchini, cleaved shallot, half teaspoon of Italian flavoring and salt and blend until vegetables are somewhat soft.
- Include chopped tomatoes, chicken stock, dry white wine and little pasta. When the pasta is soft, include spinach and cooked chicken at that point serve.

FRESH MEXICAN TUNA SALAD

Protein: 53.7 grams

Key benefits: Easy to get ready and wealthy in Omega-3 unsaturated fats (from the tuna)

Preparation:

- This is a quite simple recipe that is flawless to fulfill your craving. Apply salt in cut onions and spread it first with water to dispose of the after-taste. After soaking (in a perfect world, 30 minutes) the salted onions, channel and flush the salt.
- At that point chop the tomatoes and cilantro and blend it with the onions.
- Crush lime juice at that point add the drained tuna to the vegetable mix and delicately toss in ingredients.
- At that point make the most of your plate of vegetables. You can include organic products, for example, peeled apples or oranges on the off chance that you need to have that sweet, tart taste.

Now all you have to do is pick a specific intermittent fasting plan and work with it. The reason why the keto diet is the preferred diet is that it still helps us reduce our carb intake which means more weight loss. The next chapter would present you with many recipes from the keto diet which you can also fit into your 14-day diet plan and fast accordingly.

CHAPTER 5 - KETO COOK BOOK FOR INTERMITTENT FASTING

Here we have a 21-days meal plan just to guide you on your keto journey and what's more is that here we have directions, preparation time, serving directions cooking time as well as majority of the information that would make the keto diet much more of a variety than a burden, getting you into ketosis in style. Let's go.

DAY 1

BREAKFAST: POACHED EGGS

If you are on a Ketogenic diet, then this recipe is perfect for breakfast!

Preparation time: 10 minutes

Cooking time: 35 minutes

Servings: 4

Ingredients:

- 3 garlic cloves, minced
- 1 tablespoon ghee

- 1 white onion, chopped
- 1 Serrano pepper, chopped
- Salt and black pepper to the taste
- 1 red bell pepper, chopped
- 3 tomatoes, chopped
- 1 teaspoon paprika
- 1 teaspoon cumin
- ¼ teaspoon chili powder
- 1 tablespoon cilantro, chopped
- 6 eggs

Directions:

1. Heat up a pan with the ghee over medium heat, add onion, stir and cook for 10 minutes.
2. Add Serrano pepper and garlic, stir and cook for 1 minute.
3. Add red bell pepper, stir and cook for 10 minutes.
4. Add tomatoes, salt, pepper, chili powder, cumin and paprika, stir and cook for 10 minutes.
5. Crack eggs into the pan, season them with salt and pepper, cover pan and cook for 6 minutes more.
6. Sprinkle cilantro at the end and serve.
7. Enjoy!

Nutrition: calories 300, fat 12, fiber 3.4, carbs 22, protein 14

LUNCH: CAESAR SALAD

This is packed with healthy elements and it's 100% keto!

Preparation time: 10 minutes

Cooking time: 0 minutes

Servings: 2

Ingredients:

- 1 avocado, pitted, peeled and sliced
- Salt and black pepper to the taste
- 3 tablespoons creamy Caesar dressing
- 1 cup bacon, cooked and crumbled
- 1 chicken breast, grilled and shredded

Directions:

1. In a salad bowl, mix avocado with bacon and chicken breast and stir.
2. Add Caesar dressing, salt and pepper, toss to coat, divide into 2 bowls and serve.

Enjoy!

Nutrition: calories 334, fat 23, fiber 4, carbs 3, protein 18

DINNER: SPECIAL FISH PIE

This is really creamy and rich!

Preparation time: 10 minutes

Cooking time: 1 hour and 10 minutes

Servings: 6

Ingredients:

- 1 red onion, chopped
- 2 salmon fillets, skinless and cut into medium pieces
- 2 mackerel fillets, skinless and cut into medium pieces
- 3 haddock fillets and cut into medium pieces
- 2 bay leaves
- ¼ cup ghee+ 2 tablespoons ghee
- 1 cauliflower head, florets separated
- 4 eggs
- 4 cloves
- 1 cup whipping cream
- ½ cup water
- A pinch of nutmeg, ground
- 1 teaspoon Dijon mustard
- 1 cup cheddar cheese, shredded+ ½ cup cheddar cheese, shredded
- Some chopped parsley

- Salt and black pepper to the taste
- 4 tablespoons chives, chopped

Directions:

1. Put some water in a pan, add some salt, bring to a boil over medium heat, add eggs, , cook them for 10 minutes, take off heat, drain, leave them to cool down, peel and cut them into quarters.
2. Put water in another pot, bring to a boil, add cauliflower florets, cook for 10 minutes, drain them, transfer to your blender, add ¼ cup ghee, pulse well and transfer to a bowl.
3. Put cream and ½ cup water in a pan, add fish, toss to coat and heat up over medium heat.
4. Add onion, cloves and bay leaves, bring to a boil, reduce heat and simmer for 10 minutes.
5. Take off heat, transfer fish to a baking dish and leave aside.
6. Return pan with fish sauce to heat, add nutmeg, stir and cook for 5 minutes.
7. Take off heat, discard cloves and bay leaves, add 1 cup cheddar cheese and 2 tablespoons ghee and stir well.
8. Place egg quarters on top of the fish in the baking dish.

9. Add cream and cheese sauce over them, top with cauliflower mash, sprinkle the rest of the cheddar cheese, chives and parsley, introduce in the oven at 400 degrees F for 30 minutes.
10. Leave the pie to cool down a bit before slicing and serving.

Enjoy!

Nutrition: calories 300, fat 45, fiber 3, carbs 5, protein 26

DESSERT: CHOCOLATE TRUFFLES

These are so wonderful and delicious!

Preparation time: 10 minutes

Cooking time: 6 minutes

Servings: 22

Ingredients:

- 1 cup sugar free- chocolate chips
- 2 tablespoons butter
- 2/3 cup heavy cream
- 2 teaspoons brandy
- 2 tablespoons swerve
- ¼ teaspoon vanilla extract
- Cocoa powder

Directions:

1. Put heavy cream in a heat proof bowl, add swerve, butter and chocolate chips, stir, introduce in your microwave and heat up for 1 minute.
2. Leave aside for 5 minutes, stir well and mix with brandy and vanilla.

3. Stir again, leave aside in the fridge for a couple of hours.
4. Use a melon baller to shape your truffles, roll them in cocoa powder and serve them.

Enjoy!

Nutrition: calories 60, fat 5, fiber 4, carbs 6, protein 1

DAY 2

BREAKFAST: BREAKFAST BOWL

You will feel full of energy all day with this keto breakfast!

Preparation time: 10 minutes

Cooking time: 20 minutes

Servings: 1

Ingredients:

- 4 ounces beef, ground
- 1 yellow onion, chopped
- 8 mushrooms, sliced
- Salt and black pepper to the taste
- 2 eggs, whisked
- 1 tablespoon coconut oil
- ½ teaspoon smoked paprika
- 1 avocado, pitted, peeled and chopped
- 12 black olives, pitted and sliced

Directions:

1. Heat up a pan with the coconut oil over medium heat, add onions, mushrooms, salt and pepper, stir and cook for 5 minutes.
2. Add beef and paprika, stir, cook for 10 minutes and transfer to a bowl.
3. Heat up the pan again over medium heat, add eggs, some salt and pepper and scramble them.
4. Return beef mix to pan and stir.
5. Add avocado and olives, stir and cook for 1 minute.
6. Transfer to a bowl and serve.

Enjoy!

Nutrition: calories 600, fat 23, fiber 8, carbs 22, protein 43

LUNCH: TACOS

It's an easy and tasty lunch idea for all those who are on a Keto diet!

Preparation time: 10 minutes

Cooking time: 25 minutes

Servings: 3

Ingredients:

- 2 cups cheddar cheese, grated
- 1 small avocado, pitted, peeled and chopped
- 1 cup favorite taco meat, cooked
- 2 teaspoons sriracha sauce
- ¼ cup tomatoes, chopped
- Cooking spray
- Salt and black pepper to the taste

Directions:

1. Spray some cooking oil on lined baking dish.
2. Spread cheddar cheese on the baking sheet, introduce in the oven at 400 degrees F and bake for 15 minutes.
3. Spread taco meat over cheese and bake for 10 minutes more.

4. Meanwhile, in a bowl, mix avocado with tomatoes, sriracha sauce, salt and pepper and stir.
5. Spread this over taco and cheddar layers, leave tacos to cool down a bit, slice using a pizza slicer and serve for lunch.

Enjoy!

Nutrition: calories 400, fat 23, fiber 0, carbs 2, protein 37

DINNER: DELICIOUS CHICKEN NUGGETS

This is perfect for a friendly meal!

Preparation time: 10 minutes

Cooking time: 15 minutes

Servings: 2

Ingredients:

- ½ cup coconut flour
- 1 egg
- 2 tablespoons garlic powder
- 2 chicken breasts, cubed
- Salt and black pepper to the taste
- ½ cup ghee

Directions:

1. In a bowl, mix garlic powder with coconut flour, salt and pepper and stir.
2. In another bowl, whisk egg well.
3. Dip chicken breast cubes in egg mix, then in flour mix.
4. Heat up a pan with the ghee over medium heat, drop chicken nuggets and cook them for 5 minutes on each side.

5. Transfer to paper towels, drain grease and then serve them with some tasty ketchup on the side.

Enjoy!

Nutrition: calories 60, fat 3, fiber 0.2, carbs 3, protein 4

DESSERT: DELICIOUS DOUGHNUTS

These keto doughnuts look and taste wonderful!

Preparation time: 10 minutes

Cooking time: 15 minutes

Servings: 24

Ingredients:

- ¼ cup erythritol
- ¼ cup flaxseed meal
- ¾ cup almond flour
- 1 teaspoon baking powder
- 1 teaspoon vanilla extract
- 2 eggs
- 3 tablespoons coconut oil
- ¼ cup coconut milk
- 20 drops red food coloring
- A pinch of salt
- 1 tablespoon cocoa powder

Directions:

1. In a bowl, mix flaxseed meal with almond flour, cocoa powder, baking powder, erythritol and salt and stir.

2. In another bowl, mix coconut oil with coconut milk, vanilla, food coloring and eggs and stir.
3. Combine the 2 mixtures, stir using a hand mixer, transfer to a bag, make a hole in the bag and shape 12 doughnuts on a baking sheet.
4. Introduce in the oven at 350 degrees F and bake for 15 minutes.
5. Arrange them on a platter and serve them.

Enjoy!

Nutrition: calories 60, fat 4, fiber 0, carbs 1, protein 2

DAY3

BREAKFAST: EGGS AND SAUSAGES

Try a different keto breakfast each day! Try this one!

Preparation time: 10 minutes

Cooking time: 35 minutes

Servings: 6

Ingredients:

- 5 tablespoons ghee
- 12 eggs
- Salt and black pepper to the taste
- 1-ounce spinach, torn
- 12 ham slices
- 2 sausages, chopped
- 1 yellow onion, chopped
- 1 red bell pepper, chopped

Directions:

1. Heat up a pan with 1 tablespoon ghee over medium heat, add sausages and onion, stir and cook for 5 minutes.

2. Add bell pepper, salt and pepper, stir and cook for 3 minutes more and transfer to a bowl.
3. Melt the rest of the ghee and divide into 12 cupcake molds.
4. Add a slice of ham in each cupcake mold, divide spinach in each and then the sausage mix.
5. Crack an egg on top, introduce everything in the oven and bake at 425 degrees F for 20 minutes.
6. Leave your keto cupcakes to cool down a bit before serving.

Enjoy!

Nutrition: calories 440, fat 32, fiber 0, carbs 12, protein 22

LUNCH: PIZZA

We recommend you to try this Ketogenic pizza for lunch today!

Preparation time: 10 minutes

Cooking time: 7 minutes

Servings: 4

Ingredients:

- 1 cup pizza cheese mix, shredded
- 1 tablespoon olive oil
- 2 tablespoons ghee
- 1 cup mozzarella cheese, shredded
- ¼ cup mascarpone cheese
- 1 tablespoon heavy cream
- 1 teaspoon garlic, minced
- Salt and black pepper to the taste
- A pinch of lemon pepper
- 1/3 cup broccoli florets, steamed
- Some asiago cheese, shaved for serving

Directions:

1. Heat up a pan with the oil over medium heat, add pizza cheese mix and spread into a circle.

2. Add mozzarella cheese and also spread into a circle.
3. Cook everything for 5 minutes and transfer to a plate.
4. Heat up the pan with the ghee over medium heat, add mascarpone cheese, cream, salt, pepper, lemon pepper and garlic, stir and cook for 5 minutes.
5. Drizzle half of this mix over cheese crust.
6. Add broccoli florets to the pan with the rest of the mascarpone mix, stir and cook for 1 minute.
7. Add this on top of the pizza, sprinkle asiago cheese at the end and serve.

Enjoy!

Nutrition: calories 250, fat 15, fiber 1, carbs 3, protein 10

DINNER: BAKED FISH

It's an easy keto dish for you to enjoy tonight for dinner!

Preparation time: 10 minutes

Cooking time: 30 minutes

Servings: 4

Ingredients:

- 1-pound haddock
- 3 teaspoons water
- 2 tablespoons lemon juice
- Salt and black pepper to the taste
- 2 tablespoons mayonnaise
- 1 teaspoon dill weed
- Cooking spray
- A pinch of old bay seasoning

Directions:

1. Spray a baking dish with some cooking oil.
2. Add lemon juice, water and fish and toss to coat a bit.
3. Add salt, pepper, old bay seasoning and dill weed and toss again.
4. Add mayo and spread well.

5. Introduce in the oven at 350 degrees F and bake for 30 minutes.
6. Divide between plates and serve.

Enjoy!

Nutrition: calories 104, fat 12, fiber 1, carbs 0.5, protein 20

DESSERT: CHOCOLATE BOMBS

You must try these today!

Preparation time: 10 minutes

Cooking time: 10 minutes

Servings: 12

Ingredients:

- 10 tablespoons coconut oil
- 3 tablespoons macadamia nuts, chopped
- 2 packets stevia
- 5 tablespoons unsweetened coconut powder
- A pinch of salt

Directions:

1. Put coconut oil in a pot and melt over medium heat.
2. Add stevia, salt and cocoa powder, stir well and take off heat.
3. Spoon this into a candy tray and keep in the fridge for a while.
4. Sprinkle macadamia nuts on top and keep in the fridge until you serve them.

Enjoy!

Nutrition: calories 50, fat 1, fiber 0, carbs 1, protein 2

DAY4

BREAKFAST: SCRAMBLED EGGS

They taste delicious!

Preparation time: 10 minutes

Cooking time: 10 minutes

Servings: 1

Ingredients:

- 4 bell mushrooms, chopped
- 3 eggs, whisked
- Salt and black pepper to the taste
- 2 ham slices, chopped
- ¼ cup red bell pepper, chopped
- ½ cup spinach, chopped
- 1 tablespoon coconut oil

Directions:

1. Heat up a pan with half of the oil over medium heat, add mushrooms, spinach, ham and bell pepper, stir and cook for 4 minutes.
2. Heat up another pan with the rest of the oil over medium heat, add eggs and scramble them.

3. Add veggies and ham, salt and pepper, stir, cook for 1 minute and serve.

Enjoy!

Nutrition: calories 350, fat 23, fiber 1, carbs 5, protein 22

LUNCH: EASY DISH

Get all the ingredients you need and make this amazing keto lunch as soon as possible!

Preparation time: 10 minutes

Cooking time: 15 minutes

Servings: 2

Ingredients:

- 1 and ½ cups cheddar cheese, shredded
- 1 and ½ cups cheese blend
- 2 beef hot dogs, finely chopped
- A drizzle of olive oil
- 1 pound beef meat, ground
- Salt and black pepper to the taste
- ¼ teaspoon paprika
- ¼ teaspoon old bay
- ¼ teaspoon onion powder
- ¼ teaspoon garlic powder
- 1 cup lettuce leaves, chopped
- 1 tablespoon thousand island dressing
- 2 tablespoons dill pickle, chopped
- 2 tablespoons yellow onion, chopped
- ½ cup American cheese, shredded
- Some ketchup for serving
- Some mustard for serving

Directions:

1. Heat up a pan with a drizzle of oil over medium heat, add half of the cheese blend, spread into a circle and top with half of the cheddar cheese.
2. Also spread into a circle, cook for 5 minutes, transfer to a cutting board and leave aside for a few minutes to cool down.
3. Heat up the pan again, add the rest of the cheese blend and spread into a circle.
4. Add the rest of the cheddar, also spread, cook for 5 minutes and also transfer to a cutting board.
5. Spread the thousand island dressing over the 2 pizza crusts.
6. Heat up the same pan again over medium heat, add beef, stir and brown for a few minutes.
7. Add salt, pepper, old bay seasoning, paprika, onion and garlic powder, stir and cook for a few minutes more.
8. Add hot dogs pieces, stir and cook for 5 minutes more.
9. Spread lettuce, pickles, American cheese and onions on the 2 pizza crusts.
10. Divide beef and hot dog mix, drizzle mustard and ketchup at the end and serve.

Nutrition: calories 200, fat 6, fiber 3, carbs 1.5, protein 10

DINNER: CHICKEN WINGS AND TASTY MINT CHUTNEY

It's so fresh and delicious!

Preparation time: 20 minutes

Cooking time: 25 minutes

Servings: 6

Ingredients:

- 18 chicken wings, cut in halves
- 1 tablespoon turmeric
- 1 tablespoon cumin, ground
- 1 tablespoon ginger, grated
- 1 tablespoon coriander, ground
- 1 tablespoon paprika
- A pinch of cayenne pepper
- Salt and black pepper to the taste
- 2 tablespoons olive oil

For the chutney:

- Juice of ½ lime
- 1 cup mint leaves
- 1 small ginger piece, chopped
- ¾ cup cilantro
- 1 tablespoon olive oil
- 1 tablespoon water

- Salt and black pepper to the taste
- 1 Serrano pepper

Directions:

1. In a bowl, mix 1 tablespoon ginger with cumin, coriander, paprika, turmeric, salt, pepper, cayenne and 2 tablespoons oil and stir well.
2. Add chicken wings pieces to this mix, toss to coat well and keep in the fridge for 20 minutes.
3. Heat up your grill over high heat, add marinated wings, cook for 25 minutes, turning them from time to time and transfer to a bowl.
4. In your blender, mix mint with cilantro, 1 small ginger pieces, juice from ½ lime, 1 tablespoon olive oil, salt, pepper, water and Serrano pepper and blend very well.
5. Serve your chicken wings with this sauce on the side.

Enjoy!

Nutrition: calories 100, fat 5, fiber 1, carbs 1, protein 9

DESSERT: AMAZING JELLO DESSERT

It's more than you can imagine!

Preparation time: 2 hours 10 minutes

Cooking time: 5 minutes

Servings: 12

Ingredients:

- 2 ounces packets sugar free jello
- 1 cup cold water
- 1 cup hot water
- 3 tablespoons erythritol
- 2 tablespoons gelatin powder
- 1 teaspoon vanilla extract
- 1 cup heavy cream
- 1 cup boiling water

Directions:

1. Put jello packets in a bowl, add 1 cup hot water, stir until it dissolves and then mix with 1 cup cold water.
2. Pour this into a lined square dish and keep in the fridge for 1 hour.
3. Cut into cubes and leave aside for now.

4. Meanwhile, in a bowl, mix erythritol with vanilla extract, 1 cup boiling water, gelatin and heavy cream and stir very well.
5. Pour half of this mix into a silicon round mold, spread jello cubes, then top with the rest of the gelatin.
6. Keep in the fridge for 1 more hour and then serve.

Enjoy!

Nutrition: calories 70, fat 1, fiber 0, carbs 1, protein 2

DAY5

BREAKFAST: FRITTATA

Try a keto frittata today! It's so tasty!

Preparation time: 10 minutes

Cooking time: 1 hour

Servings: 4

Ingredients:

- 9 ounces spinach
- 12 eggs
- 1-ounce pepperoni
- 1 teaspoon garlic, minced
- Salt and black pepper to the taste
- 5 ounces mozzarella, shredded
- ½ cup parmesan, grated
- ½ cup ricotta cheese
- 4 tablespoons olive oil
- A pinch of nutmeg

Directions:

1. Squeeze liquid from spinach and put in a bowl.
2. In another bowl, mix eggs with salt, pepper, nutmeg and garlic and whisk well.
3. Add spinach, parmesan and ricotta and whisk well again.
4. Pour this into a pan, sprinkle mozzarella and pepperoni on top, introduce in the oven and bake at 375 degrees F for 45 minutes.
5. Leave frittata to cool down for a few minutes before serving it.

Enjoy!

Nutrition: calories 298, fat 2, fiber 1, carbs 6, protein 18

LUNCH: MEXICAN DREAM

It's so delicious! Why don't you try it today?

Preparation time: 10 minutes

Cooking time: 20 minutes

Servings: 4

Ingredients:

- ¼ cup cilantro, chopped
- 2 avocados, pitted, peeled and cut into chunks
- 1 tablespoon lime juice
- ¼ cup white onion, chopped
- 1 teaspoon garlic, minced
- Salt and black pepper to the taste
- 6 cherry tomatoes, cut in quarters
- ½ cup water
- 2-pound beef meat, ground
- 2 cups sour cream
- ¼ cup taco seasoning
- 2 cups lettuce leaves, shredded
- Some cayenne pepper sauce for serving
- 2 cups cheddar cheese, shredded

Directions:

1. In a bowl, mix cilantro with lime juice, avocado, onion, tomatoes, salt, pepper and garlic, stir well and leave aside in the fridge for now.
2. Heat up a pan over medium heat, add beef, stir and brown for 10 minutes.
3. Add taco seasoning and water, stir and cook over medium-low heat for 10 minutes more.
4. Divide this mix into 4 serving bowls.
5. Add sour cream, avocado mix you've made earlier, lettuce pieces and cheddar cheese.
6. Drizzle cayenne pepper sauce at the end and serve for lunch!

Enjoy!

Nutrition: calories 340, fat 30, fiber 5, carbs 3, protein 32

DINNER: TILAPIA

This great dish is perfect for a special evening!

Preparation time: 10 minutes

Cooking time: 10 minutes

Servings: 4

Ingredients:

- 4 tilapia fillets, boneless
- Salt and black pepper to the taste
- ½ cup parmesan, grated
- 4 tablespoons mayonnaise
- ¼ teaspoon basil, dried
- ¼ teaspoon garlic powder
- 2 tablespoons lemon juice
- ¼ cup ghee
- Cooking spray
- A pinch of onion powder

Directions:

1. Spray a baking sheet with cooking spray, place tilapia on it, season with salt and pepper, introduce in preheated broiler and cook for 3 minutes.
2. Turn fish on the other side and broil for 3 minutes more.

3. In a bowl, mix parmesan with mayo, basil, garlic, lemon juice, onion powder and ghee and stir well.
4. Add fish to this mix, toss to coat well, place on baking sheet again and broil for 3 minutes more.
5. Transfer to plates and serve.

Enjoy!

Nutrition: calories 175, fat 10, fiber 0, carbs 2, protein 17

DESSERT: MUG CAKE

This is very simple and tasty!

Preparation time: 2 minutes

Cooking time: 3 minutes

Servings: 1

Ingredients:

- 4 tablespoons almond meal
- 2 tablespoon ghee
- 1 teaspoon stevia
- 1 tablespoon cocoa powder, unsweetened
- 1 egg
- 1 tablespoon coconut flour
- ¼ teaspoon vanilla extract
- ½ teaspoon baking powder

Directions:

1. Put the ghee in a mug and introduce in the microwave for a couple of seconds.
2. Add cocoa powder, stevia, egg, baking powder, vanilla and coconut flour and stir well.
3. Add almond meal as well, stir again, introduce in the microwave and cook for 2 minutes.
4. Serve your mug cake with berries on top.

Enjoy!

Nutrition: calories 450, fat 34, fiber 7, carbs 10, protein 20

DAY 6

BREAKFAST: SMOKED SALMON BREAKFAST

It will surprise you with its taste!

Preparation time: 10 minutes

Cooking time: 10 minutes

Servings: 3

Ingredients:

- 4 eggs, whisked
- ½ teaspoon avocado oil
- 4 ounces smoked salmon, chopped
- For the sauce:
- 1 cup coconut milk
- ½ cup cashews, soaked, drained
- ¼ cup green onions, chopped
- 1 teaspoon garlic powder
- Salt and black pepper to the taste
- 1 tablespoon lemon juice

Directions:

1. In your blender, mix cashews with coconut milk, garlic powder and lemon juice and blend well.

2. Add salt, pepper and green onions, blend again well, transfer to a bowl and keep in the fridge for now.
3. Heat up a pan with the oil over medium-low heat, add eggs, whisk a bit and cook until they are almost done
4. Introduce in your preheated broiler and cook until eggs set.
5. Divide eggs on plates, top with smoked salmon and serve with the green onion sauce on top.

Enjoy!

Nutrition: calories 200, fat 10, fiber 2, carbs 11, protein 15

LUNCH: STUFFED PEPPERS

These are perfect for a Ketogenic lunch!

Preparation time: 10 minutes

Cooking time: 40 minutes

Servings: 4

Ingredients:

- 4 big banana peppers, tops cut off, seeds removed and cut into halves lengthwise
- 1 tablespoon ghee
- Salt and black pepper to the taste
- ½ teaspoon herbs de Provence
- 1 pound sweet sausage, chopped
- 3 tablespoons yellow onions, chopped
- Some marinara sauce
- A drizzle of olive oil

Directions:

1. Season banana peppers with salt and pepper, drizzle the oil, rub well and bake in the oven at 350 degrees F for 20 minutes.
2. Meanwhile, heat up a pan over medium heat, add sausage pieces, stir and cook for 5 minutes.
3. Add onion, herbs de Provence, salt, pepper and ghee, stir well and cook for 5 minutes.

4. Take peppers out of the oven, fill them with the sausage mix, place them in an oven-proof dish, drizzle marinara sauce over them, introduce in the oven again and bake for 10 minutes more.
5. Serve hot.

Enjoy!

Nutrition: calories 320, fat 8, fiber 4, carbs 3, protein 10

DINNER: CHICKEN MEATBALLS

Hurry up and make these amazing meatballs today!

Preparation time: 10 minutes

Cooking time: 15 minutes

Servings: 3

Ingredients:

- 1-pound chicken meat, ground
- Salt and black pepper to the taste
- 2 tablespoons ranch dressing
- ½ cup almond flour
- ¼ cup cheddar cheese, grated
- 1 tablespoon dry ranch seasoning
- ¼ cup hot sauce+ some more for serving
- 1 egg

Directions:

1. In a bowl, mix chicken meat with salt, pepper, ranch dressing, flour, dry ranch seasoning, cheddar cheese, hot sauce and the egg and Stir very well.
2. Shape 9 meatballs, place them all on a lined baking sheet and bake at 500 degrees F for 15 minutes.

3. Serve chicken meatballs with hot sauce on the side.

Enjoy!

Nutrition: calories 156, fat 11, fiber 1, carbs 2, protein 12

DESSERT: STRAWBERRY PIE

It's so delicious!

Preparation time: 2 hours and 10 minutes

Cooking time: 5 minutes

Servings: 12

Ingredients:

For the crust:

- 1 cup coconut, shredded
- 1 cup sunflower seeds
- ¼ cup butter
- A pinch of salt

For the filling:

- 1 teaspoon gelatin
- 8 ounces cream cheese
- 4 ounces strawberries
- 2 tablespoons water
- ½ tablespoon lemon juice
- ¼ teaspoon stevia
- ½ cup heavy cream
- 8 ounces strawberries, chopped for serving
- 16 ounces heavy cream for serving

Directions:

1. In your food processor, mix sunflower seeds with coconut, a pinch of salt and butter and stir well.
2. Put this into a greased spring form pan and press well on the bottom.
3. Heat up a pan with the water over medium heat, add gelatin, stir until it dissolves, take off heat and leave aside to cool down.
4. Add this to your food processor, mix with 4 ounces strawberries, cream cheese, lemon juice and stevia and blend well.
5. Add ½ cup heavy cream, stir well and spread this over crust.
6. Top with 8 ounces strawberries and 16 ounces heavy cream and keep in the fridge for 2 hours before slicing and serving.

Enjoy!

Nutrition: calories 234, fat 23, fiber 2, carbs 6, protein 7

DAY7

BREAKFAST: FETA & ASPARAGUS

These elements combine very well!

Preparation time: 10 minutes

Cooking time: 25 minutes

Servings: 2

Ingredients:

- 12 asparagus spears
- 1 tablespoon olive oil
- 2 green onions, chopped
- 1 garlic clove, minced
- 6 eggs
- Salt and black pepper to the taste
- ½ cup feta cheese

Directions:

1. Heat up a pan with some water over medium heat, add asparagus, cook for 8 minutes, drain well, chop 2 spears and reserve the rest.
2. Heat up a pan with the oil over medium heat, add garlic, chopped asparagus and onions, stir and cook for 5 minutes.

3. Add eggs, salt and pepper, stir, cover and cook for 5 minutes.
4. Arrange the whole asparagus on top of your frittata, sprinkle cheese, introduce in the oven at 350 degrees F and bake for 9 minutes.
5. Divide between plates and serve.

Enjoy!

Nutrition: calories 340, fat 12, fiber 3, carbs 8, protein 26

LUNCH: BURGERS

These burgers are really something very special!

Preparation time: 10 minutes

Cooking time: 25 minutes

Servings: 8

Ingredients:

- 1 pound brisket, ground
- 1 pound beef, ground
- Salt and black pepper to the taste
- 8 butter slices
- 1 tablespoon garlic, minced
- 1 tablespoon Italian seasoning
- 2 tablespoons mayonnaise
- 1 tablespoon ghee
- 2 tablespoons olive oil
- 1 yellow onion, chopped
- 1 tablespoon water

Directions:

1. In a bowl, mix brisket with beef, salt, pepper, Italian seasoning, garlic and mayo and stir well.
2. Shape 8 patties and make a pocket in each.
3. Stuff each burger with a butter slice and seal.

4. Heat up a pan with the olive oil over medium heat, add onions, stir and cook for 2 minutes.
5. Add the water, stir and gather them in the corner of the pan.
6. Place burgers in the pan with the onions and cook them over medium-low heat for 10 minutes.
7. Flip them, add the ghee and cook them for 10 minutes more.
8. Divide burgers on buns and serve them with caramelized onions on top.

Enjoy!

Nutrition: calories 180, fat 8, fiber 1, carbs 4, protein 20

DINNER: TROUT & SPECIAL SAUCE

You just have to try this wonderful combination! This keto dish is great!

Preparation time: 10 minutes

Cooking time: 10 minutes

Servings: 1

Ingredients:

- 1 big trout fillet
- Salt and black pepper to the taste
- 1 tablespoon olive oil
- 1 tablespoon ghee
- Zest and juice from 1 orange
- A handful parsley, chopped
- ½ cup pecans, chopped

Directions:

1. Heat up a pan with the oil over medium high heat, add the fish fillet, season with salt and pepper, cook for 4 minutes on each side, transfer to a plate and keep warm for now.
2. Heat up the same pan with the ghee over medium heat, add pecans, stir and toast for 1 minutes.

3. Add orange juice and zest, some salt and pepper and chopped parsley, stir, cook for 1 minute and pour over fish fillet.
4. Serve right away.

Enjoy!

Nutrition: calories 200, fat 10, fiber 2, carbs 1, protein 14

DESSERT: VANILLA PARFAITS

These will make you feel amazing!

Preparation time: 10 minutes

Cooking time: 0 minutes

Servings: 4

Ingredients:

- 14 ounces canned coconut milk
- 1 teaspoon vanilla extract
- 10 drops stevia
- 4 ounces berries
- 2 tablespoons walnuts, chopped

Directions:

1. In a bowl, mix coconut milk with stevia and vanilla extract and whisk using your mixer.
2. IN another bowl, mix berries with walnuts and stir.
3. Spoon half of vanilla coconut mix into 4 jars, add a layer of berries and top with the rest of the vanilla mix.
4. Top with berries and walnuts mix, introduce in the fridge until you serve it.

Enjoy!

Nutrition: calories 400, fat 23, fiber 4, carbs 6, protein 7

DAY 8

BREAKFAST: SPECIAL EGGS

This is truly the best keto eggs recipe you can ever try!

Preparation time: 10 minutes

Cooking time: 4 minutes

Servings: 12

Ingredients:

- 4 tea bags
- 4 tablespoons salt
- 12 eggs
- 2 tablespoons cinnamon
- 6-star anise
- 1 teaspoon black pepper
- 1 tablespoon peppercorn
- 8 cups water
- 1 cup tamari sauce

Directions:

1. Put water in a pot, add eggs, bring them to a boil over medium heat and cook until they are hard boiled.
2. Cool them down and crack them without peeling.
3. In a large pot, mix water with tea bags, salt, pepper, peppercorns, cinnamon, star anise and tamari sauce.
4. Add cracked eggs, cover pot, bring to a simmer over low heat and cook for 30 minutes.
5. Discard tea bags and cook eggs for 3 hours and 30 minutes.
6. Leave eggs to cool down, peel and serve them for breakfast.

Enjoy!

Nutrition: calories 90, fat 6, fiber 0, carbs 0, protein 7

LUNCH: ZUCCHINI DISH

It's easy to make and very light! Try this lunch dish soon!

Preparation time: 10 minutes

Cooking time: 5 minutes

Servings: 1

Ingredients:

- 1 tablespoon olive oil
- 3 tablespoons ghee
- 2 cups zucchini, cut with a spiralizer
- 1 teaspoon red pepper flakes
- 1 tablespoon garlic, minced
- 1 tablespoon red bell pepper, chopped
- Salt and black pepper to the taste
- 1 tablespoon basil, chopped
- ¼ cup asiago cheese, shaved
- ¼ cup parmesan, grated

Directions:

1. Heat up a pan with the oil and ghee over medium heat, add garlic, bell pepper and pepper flakes, stir and cook for 1 minute.

2. Add zucchini noodles, stir and cook for 2 minutes more.
3. Add basil, parmesan, salt and pepper, stir and cook for a few seconds more.
4. Take off heat, transfer to a bowl and serve for lunch with asiago cheese on top.

Enjoy!

Nutrition: calories 140, fat 3, fiber 1, carbs 1.3, protein 5

DINNER: GRILLED CHICKEN WINGS

You will have these done in no time and they will taste wonderful!

Preparation time: 2 hours and 10 minutes

Cooking time: 15 minutes

Servings: 5

Ingredients:

- 2 pounds wings
- Juice from 1 lime
- 1 handful cilantro, chopped
- 2 garlic cloves, minced
- 1 jalapeno pepper, chopped
- 3 tablespoons coconut oil
- Salt and black pepper to the taste
- Lime wedges for serving
- Ranch dip for serving

Directions:

1. In a bowl, mix lime juice with cilantro, garlic, jalapeno, coconut oil, salt and pepper and whisk well.

2. Add chicken wings, toss to coat and keep in the fridge for 2 hours.
3. Place chicken wings on your preheated grill over medium high heat and cook for 7 minutes on each side.
4. Serve these amazing chicken wings with ranch did and lime wedges on the side.

Enjoy!

Nutrition: calories 132, fat 5, fiber 1, carbs 4, protein 12

DESSERT: DELICIOUS CHOCOLATE PIE

This special pie will impress your loved ones for sure!

Preparation time: 3 hours 10 minutes

Cooking time: 20 minutes

Servings: 10

Ingredients:

For the crust:

- ½ teaspoon baking powder
- 1 and ½ cup almond crust
- A pinch of salt
- 1/3 cup stevia
- 1 egg
- 1 and ½ teaspoons vanilla extract
- 3 tablespoons butter
- 1 teaspoon butter for the pan

For the filling:

- 1 tablespoon vanilla extract
- 4 tablespoons butter
- 4 tablespoons sour cream
- 16 ounces cream cheese

- ½ cup cut stevia
- ½ cup cocoa powder
- 2 teaspoons granulated stevia
- 1 cup whipping cream
- 1 teaspoon vanilla extract

Directions:

1. Grease a spring form pan with 1 teaspoon butter and leave aside for now.
2. In a bowl, mix baking powder with 1/3 cup stevia, a pinch of salt and almond flour and stir.
3. Add 3 tablespoons butter, egg and 1 and ½ teaspoon vanilla extract, stir until you obtain a dough.
4. Press this well into spring form pan, introduce in the oven at 375 degrees F and bake for 11 minutes.
5. Take pie crust out of the oven, cover with tin foil and bake for 8 minutes more.
6. Take it again out of the oven and leave it aside to cool down.
7. Meanwhile, in a bowl, mix cream cheese with 4 tablespoons butter, sour cream, 1 tablespoon vanilla extract, cocoa powder and ½ cup stevia and stir well.
8. In another bowl, mix whipping cream with 2 teaspoons stevia and 1 teaspoon vanilla extract and stir using your mixer.

9. Combine the 2 mixtures, pour into pie crust, spread well, introduce in the fridge for 3 hours and then serve.

Nutrition: calories 450, fat 43, fiber 3, carbs 7, protein 7

DAY 9

BREAKFAST: EGGS BAKED IN AVOCADOS

They are so delicious and they look great too!

Preparation time: 10 minutes

Cooking time: 20 minutes

Servings: 4

Ingredients:

- 2 avocados, cut in halves and pitted
- 4 eggs
- Salt and black pepper to the taste
- 1 tablespoon chives, chopped

Directions:

1. Scoop some flesh from the avocado halves and arrange them in a baking dish.
2. Crack an egg in each avocado, season with salt and pepper, introduce them in the oven at 425 degrees F and bake for 20 minutes.
3. Sprinkle chives at the end and serve for breakfast!

Enjoy!

Nutrition: calories 400, fat 34, fiber 13, carbs 13, protein 15

LUNCH: BACON & ZUCCHINI NOODLES SALAD

It's so refreshing and healthy! We adore this salad!

Preparation time: 10 minutes

Cooking time: 0 minutes

Servings: 2

Ingredients:

- 1 cup baby spinach
- 4 cups zucchini noodles
- 1/3 cup bleu cheese, crumbled
- 1/3 cup thick cheese dressing
- ½ cup bacon, cooked and crumbled
- Black pepper to the taste

Directions:

1. In a salad bowl, mix spinach with zucchini noodles, bacon and bleu cheese and toss.
2. Add cheese dressing and black pepper to the taste, toss well to coat, divide into 2 bowls and serve.

Enjoy!

Virginia Cooke

Nutrition: calories 200, fat 14, fiber 4, carbs 2, protein 10

DINNER: TROUT AND GHEE SAUCE

The fish goes so well with the sauce! You have to try today!

Preparation time: 10 minutes

Cooking time: 10 minutes

Servings: 4

Ingredients:

- 4 trout fillets
- Salt and black pepper to the taste
- 3 teaspoons lemon zest, grated
- 3 tablespoons chives, chopped
- 6 tablespoons ghee
- 2 tablespoons olive oil
- 2 teaspoons lemon juice

Directions:

1. Season trout with salt and pepper, drizzle the olive oil and massage a bit.
2. Heat up your kitchen grill over medium high heat, add fish fillets, cook for 4 minutes, flip and cook for 4 minutes more.

3. Meanwhile, heat up a pan with the ghee over medium heat, add salt, pepper, chives, lemon juice and zest and stir well.
4. Divide fish fillets on plates, drizzle the ghee sauce over them and serve.

Enjoy!

Nutrition: calories 320, fat 12, fiber 1, carbs 2, protein 24

DESSERT: TASTY CHEESECAKES

This is a keto friendly dessert idea you must try!

Preparation time: 10 minutes

Cooking time: 15 minutes

Servings: 9

Ingredients:

For the cheesecakes:

- 2 tablespoons butter
- 8 ounces cream cheese
- 3 tablespoons coffee
- 3 eggs
- 1/3 cup swerve
- 1 tablespoon caramel syrup, sugar free

For the frosting:

- 3 tablespoons caramel syrup, sugar free
- 3 tablespoons butter
- 8 ounces mascarpone cheese, soft
- 2 tablespoons swerve

Directions:

1. In your blender, mix cream cheese with eggs, 2 tablespoons butter, coffee, 1 tablespoon caramel syrup and 1/3 cup swerve and pulse very well.
2. Spoon this into a cupcakes pan, introduce in the oven at 350 degrees F and bake for 15 minutes.
3. Leave aside to cool down and then keep in the freezer for 3 hours.
4. Meanwhile, in a bowl, mix 3 tablespoons butter with 3 tablespoons caramel syrup, 2 tablespoons swerve and mascarpone cheese and blend well.
5. Spoon these over cheesecakes and serve them.

Enjoy!

Nutrition: calories 254, fat 23, fiber 0, carbs 1, protein 5

DAY10

BREAKFAST: SHRIMP & BACON

This is a perfect breakfast idea!

Preparation time: 10 minutes

Cooking time: 15 minutes

Servings: 4

Ingredients:

- 1 cup mushrooms, sliced
- 4 bacon slices, chopped
- 4 ounces smoked salmon, chopped
- 4 ounces shrimp, deveined
- Salt and black pepper to the taste
- ½ cup coconut cream

Directions:

1. Heat up a pan over medium heat, add bacon, stir and cook for 5 minutes.
2. Add mushrooms, stir and cook for 5 minutes more.
3. Add salmon, stir and cook for 3 minutes.

4. Add shrimp and cook for 2 minutes.
5. Add salt, pepper and coconut cream, stir, cook for 1 minute, take off heat and divide between plates.

Enjoy!

Nutrition: calories 340, fat 23, fiber 1, carbs 4, protein 17

LUNCH: CHICKEN SALAD

The best chicken salad you could taste is now available for you!

Preparation time: 10 minutes

Cooking time: 0 minutes

Servings: 3

Ingredients:

- 1 green onion, chopped
- 1 celery rib, chopped
- 1 egg, hard-boiled, peeled and chopped
- 5 ounces chicken breast, roasted and chopped
- 2 tablespoons parsley, chopped
- ½ tablespoons dill relish
- Salt and black pepper to the taste
- 1/3 cup mayonnaise
- A pinch of granulated garlic
- 1 teaspoon mustard

Directions:

1. In your food processor, mix parsley with onion and celery and pulse well.

2. Transfer these to a bowl and leave aside for now.
3. Put chicken meat in your food processor, blend well and add to the bowl with the veggies.
4. Add egg pieces, salt and pepper and stir.
5. Also add mustard, mayo, dill relish and granulated garlic, toss to coat and serve right away.

Enjoy!

Nutrition: calories 283, fat 23, fiber 5, carbs 3, protein 12

DINNER: BAKED CHICKEN

It's a very simple keto chicken recipe!

Preparation time: 10 minutes

Cooking time: 20 minutes

Servings: 4

Ingredients:

- 4 bacon strips
- 4 chicken breasts
- 3 green onions, chopped
- 4 ounces ranch dressing
- 1-ounce coconut aminos
- 2 tablespoons coconut oil
- 4 ounces cheddar cheese, grated

Directions:

1. Heat up a pan with the oil over high heat, add chicken breasts, cook for 7 minutes, flip and cook for 7 more minutes.
2. Meanwhile, heat up another pan over medium high heat, add bacon, cook until it's crispy, transfer to paper towels, drain grease and crumble.

3. Transfer chicken breast to a baking dish, add coconut aminos, crumbled bacon, cheese and green onions on top, introduce in your oven, set on broiler and cook at a high temperature for 5 minutes more.
4. Divide between plates and serve hot.

Enjoy!

Nutrition: calories 450, fat 24, fiber 0, carbs 3, protein 60

DESSERT: RASPBERRY AND COCONUT DESSERT

They are easy to make and they taste delicious!

Preparation time: 10 minutes

Cooking time: 5 minutes

Servings: 12

Ingredients:

- ½ cup coconut butter
- ½ cup coconut oil
- ½ cup raspberries, dried
- ¼ cup swerve
- ½ cup coconut, shredded

Directions:

1. In your food processor, blend dried berries very well.
2. Heat up a pan with the butter over medium heat.
3. Add oil, coconut and swerve, stir and cook for 5 minutes.
4. Pour half of this into a lined baking pan and spread well.
5. Add raspberry powder and also spread.

6. Top with the rest of the butter mix, spread and keep in the fridge for a while.
7. Cut into pieces and serve.

Enjoy!

Nutrition: calories 234, fat 22, fiber 2, carbs 4, protein 2

DAY11

BREAKFAST: MEXICAN BREAKFAST

Try a Ketogenic Mexican breakfast today!

Preparation time: 10 minutes

Cooking time: 30 minutes

Servings: 8

Ingredients:

- ½ cup enchilada sauce
- 1-pound pork, ground
- 1-pound chorizo, chopped
- Salt and black pepper to the taste
- 8 eggs
- 1 tomato, chopped
- 3 tablespoons ghee
- ½ cup red onion, chopped
- 1 avocado, pitted, peeled and chopped

Directions:

1. In a bowl, mix pork with chorizo, stir and spread on a lined baking form.

2. Spread enchilada sauce on top, introduce in the oven at 350 degrees F and bake for 20 minutes.
3. Heat up a pan with the ghee over medium heat, add eggs and scramble them well.
4. Take pork mix out of the oven and spread scrambled eggs over them.
5. Sprinkle salt, pepper, tomato, onion and avocado, divide between plates and serve.

Enjoy!

Nutrition: calories 400, fat 32, fiber 4, carbs 7, protein 25

LUNCH: STEAK SALAD

If you are not in the mood for a Ketogenic chicken salad, then try a steak one instead!

Preparation time: 10 minutes

Cooking time: 20 minutes

Servings: 4

Ingredients:

- 1 and ½ pound steak, thinly sliced
- 3 tablespoons avocado oil
- Salt and black pepper to the taste
- ¼ cup balsamic vinegar
- 6 ounces sweet onion, chopped
- 1 lettuce head, chopped
- 2 garlic cloves, minced
- 4 ounces mushrooms, sliced
- 1 avocado, pitted, peeled and sliced
- 3 ounces sun-dried tomatoes, chopped
- 1 yellow bell pepper, sliced
- 1 orange bell pepper, sliced
- 1 teaspoon Italian seasoning
- 1 teaspoon red pepper flakes
- 1 teaspoon onion powder

Directions:

1. In a bowl, mix steak pieces with some salt, pepper and balsamic vinegar, toss to coat and leave aside for now.
2. Heat up a pan with the avocado oil over medium-low heat, add mushrooms, garlic, salt, pepper and onion, stir and cook for 20 minutes.
3. In a bowl, mix lettuce leaves with orange and yellow bell pepper, sun dried tomatoes and avocado and stirred.
4. Season steak pieces with onion powder, pepper flakes and Italian seasoning.
5. Place steak pieces in a broiling pan, introduce in preheated broiler and cook for 5 minutes.
6. Divide steak pieces on plates, add lettuce and avocado salad on the side and top everything with onion and mushroom mix.

Enjoy!

Nutrition: calories 435, fat 23, fiber 7, carbs 10, protein 35

DINNER: ROASTED SALMON

Feel free to serve this for a special occasion!

Preparation time: 10 minutes

Cooking time: 12 minutes

Servings: 4

Ingredients:

- 2 tablespoons ghee, soft
- 1 and ¼ pound salmon fillet
- 2 ounces Kimchi, finely chopped
- Salt and black pepper to the taste

Directions:

1. In your food processor, mix ghee with Kimchi and blend well.
2. Rub salmon with salt, pepper and Kimchi mix and place into a baking dish.
3. Introduce in the oven at 425 degrees F and bake for 15 minutes.
4. Divide between plates and serve with a side salad.

Enjoy!

Nutrition: calories 200, fat 12, fiber 0, carbs 3, protein 21

DESSERT: TASTY CHOCOLATE CUPS

Everyone will adore these chocolate delights!

Preparation time: 30 minutes

Cooking time: 5 minutes

Servings: 20

Ingredients:

- ½ cup coconut butter
- ½ cup coconut oil
- 3 tablespoons swerve
- ½ cup coconut, shredded
- 1.5-ounce cocoa butter
- 1 ounce chocolate, unsweetened
- ¼ cup cocoa powder
- ¼ teaspoon vanilla extract
- ¼ cup swerve

Directions:

1. In a pan, mix coconut butter with coconut oil, stir and heat up over medium heat.
2. Add coconut and 3 tablespoons swerve, stir well, take off heat, scoop into a lined muffin pan and keep in the fridge for 30 minutes.

3. Meanwhile, in a bowl, mix cocoa butter with chocolate, vanilla extract and ¼ cup swerve and stir well.
4. Place this over a bowl filled with boiling water and stir until everything is smooth.
5. Spoon this over coconut cupcakes, keep in the fridge for 15 minutes more and then serve.

Enjoy!

Nutrition: calories 240, fat 23, fiber 4, carbs 5, protein 2

DAY 12

BREAKFAST: PIE

Pay attention and learn how to make this great breakfast in no time!

Preparation time: 10 minutes

Cooking time: 45 minutes

Servings: 8

Ingredients:

- ½ onion, chopped
- 1 pie crust
- ½ red bell pepper, chopped
- ¾ pound beef, ground
- Salt and black pepper to the taste
- 3 tablespoons taco seasoning
- A handful cilantro, chopped
- 8 eggs
- 1 teaspoon coconut oil
- 1 teaspoon baking soda
- Mango salsa for serving

Directions:

1. Heat up a pan with the oil over medium heat, add beef, cook until it browns and mixes with salt, pepper and taco seasoning.
2. Stir again, transfer to a bowl and leave aside for now.
3. Heat up the pan again over medium heat with cooking juices from the meat, add onion and bell pepper, stir and cook for 4 minutes.
4. Add eggs, baking soda and some salt and stir well.
5. Add cilantro, stir again and take off heat.
6. Spread beef mix in pie crust, add veggies mix and spread over meat, introduce in the oven at 350 degrees F and bake for 45 minutes.
7. Leave the pie to cool down a bit, slice, divide between plates and serve with mango salsa on top.

Enjoy!

Nutrition: calories 198, fat 11, fiber 1, carbs 12, protein 12

LUNCH: FENNEL & CHICKEN SALAD

Try each day a different lunch salad! Today, we suggest you try this fennel and chicken delight!

Preparation time: 10 minutes

Cooking time: 0 minutes

Servings: 4

Ingredients:

- 3 chicken breasts, boneless, skinless, cooked and chopped
- 2 tablespoons walnut oil
- ¼ cup walnuts, toasted and chopped
- 1 and ½ cup fennel, chopped
- 2 tablespoons lemon juice
- ¼ cup mayonnaise
- 2 tablespoons fennel fronds, chopped
- Salt and black pepper to the taste
- A pinch of cayenne pepper

Directions:

1. In a bowl, mix fennel with chicken and walnuts and stir.
2. In another bowl, mix mayo with salt, pepper, fennel fronds, walnut oil, lemon juice, cayenne and garlic and stir well.

3. Pour this over chicken and fennel mix, toss to coat well and keep in the fridge until you serve.

Enjoy!

Nutrition: calories 200, fat 10, fiber 1, carbs 3, protein 7

DINNER: ITALIAN CHICKEN

This is an Italian style keto dish we really appreciate!

Preparation time: 10 minutes

Cooking time: 20 minutes

Servings: 4

Ingredients:

- ¼ cup olive oil
- 1 red onion, chopped
- 4 chicken breasts, skinless and boneless
- 4 garlic cloves, minced
- Salt and black pepper to the taste
- ½ cup Italian olives, pitted and chopped
- 4 anchovy fillets, chopped
- 1 tablespoon capers, chopped
- 1-pound tomatoes, chopped
- ½ teaspoon red chili flakes

Directions:

1. Season chicken with salt and pepper and rub with half of the oil.
2. Place into a pan which you've heated over high temperature, cook for 2 minutes, flip and cook for 2 minutes more.

3. Introduce chicken breasts in the oven at 450 degrees F and bake for 8 minutes.
4. Take chicken out of the oven and divide between plates.
5. Heat up the same pan with the rest of the oil over medium heat, add capers, onion, garlic, olives, anchovies, chili flakes and capers, stir and cook for 1 minute.
6. Add salt, pepper and tomatoes, stir and cook for 2 minutes more.
7. Drizzle this over chicken breasts and serve.

Enjoy!

Nutrition: calories 400, fat 20, fiber 1, carbs 2, protein 7

DESSERT: SIMPLE AND DELICIOUS MOUSSE

This is just hypnotizing! It's great!

Preparation time: 10 minutes

Cooking time: 0 minutes

Servings: 12

Ingredients:

- 8 ounces mascarpone cheese
- ¾ teaspoon vanilla stevia
- 1 cup whipping cream
- ½ pint blueberries
- ½ pint strawberries

Directions:

1. In a bowl, mix whipping cream with stevia and mascarpone and blend well using your mixer.
2. Arrange a layer of blueberries and strawberries in 12 glasses, then a layer of cream and so on.
3. Serve this mousse cold!

Enjoy!

Nutrition: calories 143, fat 12, fiber 1, carbs 3, protein 2

DAY 13

BREAKFAST: STIR FRY

We recommend you try this keto breakfast as soon as possible!

Preparation time: 10 minutes

Cooking time: 30 minutes

Servings: 2

Ingredients:

- ½ pounds beef meat, minced
- 2 teaspoons red chili flakes
- 1 tablespoon tamari sauce
- 2 bell peppers, chopped
- 1 teaspoon chili powder
- 1 tablespoon coconut oil
- Salt and black pepper to the taste

For the bok choy:

- 6 bunches bok choy, trimmed and chopped
- 1 teaspoon ginger, grated
- Salt to the taste

- 1 tablespoon coconut oil

For the eggs:

- 1 tablespoon coconut oil
- 2 eggs

Directions:

1. Heat up a pan with 1 tablespoon coconut oil over medium high heat, add beef and bell peppers, stir and cook for 10 minutes.
2. Add salt, pepper, tamari sauce, chili flakes and chili powder, stir, cook for 4 minutes more and take off heat.
3. Heat up another pan with 1 tablespoon oil over medium heat, add bok choy, stir and cook for 3 minutes.
4. Add salt and ginger, stir, cook for 2 minutes more and take off heat.
5. Heat up the third pan with 1 tablespoon oil over medium heat, crack eggs and fry them.
6. Divide beef and bell peppers mix into 2 bowls.
7. Divide bok choy and top with eggs.

Enjoy!

Nutrition: calories 248, fat 14, fiber 4, carbs 10, protein 14

LUNCH: STUFFED AVOCADO

It's so easy to make for lunch!

Preparation time: 10 minutes

Cooking time: 0 minutes

Servings: 1

Ingredients:

- 1 avocado
- 4 ounces canned sardines, drained
- 1 spring onion, chopped
- 1 tablespoon mayonnaise
- 1 tablespoon lemon juice
- Salt and black pepper to the taste
- ¼ teaspoon turmeric powder

Directions:

1. Cut avocado in halves, scoop flesh and put in a bowl.
2. Mash with a fork and mix with sardines.
3. Mash again with your fork and mix with onion, lemon juice, turmeric powder, salt, pepper and mayo.
4. Stir everything and divide into avocado halves.

5. Serve for lunch right away.

Enjoy!

Nutrition: calories 230, fat 34, fiber 12, carbs 5, protein 27

DINNER: SALMON MEATBALLS

Combine these tasty salmon meatballs with a Dijon sauce and enjoy!

Preparation time: 10 minutes

Cooking time: 30 minutes

Servings: 4

Ingredients:

- 2 tablespoons ghee
- 2 garlic cloves, minced
- 1/3 cup onion, chopped
- 1 pound wild salmon, boneless and minced
- ¼ cup chives, chopped
- 1 egg
- 2 tablespoons Dijon mustard
- 1 tablespoon coconut flour
- Salt and black pepper to the taste

For the sauce:

- 4 garlic cloves, minced
- 2 tablespoons ghee
- 2 tablespoons Dijon mustard
- Juice and zest of 1 lemon

- 2 cups coconut cream
- 2 tablespoons chives, chopped

Directions:

1. Heat up a pan with 2 tablespoons ghee over medium heat, add onion and 2 garlic cloves, stir, cook for 3 minutes and transfer to a bowl.
2. In another bowl, mix onion and garlic with salmon, chives, coconut flour, salt, pepper, 2 tablespoons mustard and egg and stir well.
3. Shape meatballs from the salmon mix, place on a baking sheet, introduce in the oven at 350 degrees F and bake for 25 minutes.
4. Meanwhile, heat up a pan with 2 tablespoons ghee over medium heat, add 4 garlic cloves, stir and cook for 1 minute.
5. Add coconut cream, 2 tablespoons Dijon mustard, lemon juice and zest and chives, stir and cook for 3 minutes.
6. Take salmon meatballs out of the oven, drop them into the Dijon sauce, toss, cook for 1 minute and take off heat.
7. Divide into bowls and serve.

Enjoy!

Nutrition: calories 171, fat 5, fiber 1, carbs 6, protein 23

DESSERT: SIMPLE PEANUT BUTTER FUDGE

You only need a few ingredients to make this tasty keto dessert!

Preparation time: 2 hours and 10 minutes

Cooking time: 2 minutes

Servings: 12

Ingredients:

- 1 cup peanut butter, unsweetened
- ¼ cup almond milk
- 2 teaspoons vanilla stevia
- 1 cup coconut oil
- A pinch of salt

For the topping:

- 2 tablespoons swerve
- 2 tablespoons melted coconut oil
- ¼ cup cocoa powder

Directions:

1. In a heat proof bowl, mix peanut butter with 1 cup coconut oil, stir and heat up in your microwave until it melts.
2. Add a pinch of salt, almond milk and stevia, stir well everything and pour into a lined loaf pan.
3. Keep in the fridge for 2 hours and then slice it.
4. In a bowl, mix 2 tablespoons melted coconut with cocoa powder and swerve and stir very well.
5. Drizzle the sauce over your peanut butter fudge and serve.

Enjoy!

Nutrition: calories 265, fat 23, fiber 2, carbs 4, protein 6

DAY14

BREAKFAST: SKILLET

It's going to be so tasty!

Preparation time: 10 minutes

Cooking time: 30 minutes

Servings: 4

Ingredients:

- 8 ounces mushrooms, chopped
- Salt and black pepper to the taste
- 1-pound pork, minced
- 1 tablespoon coconut oil
- ½ teaspoon garlic powder
- ½ teaspoon basil, dried
- 2 tablespoons Dijon mustard
- 2 zucchinis, chopped

Directions:

1. Heat up a pan with the oil over medium high heat, add mushrooms, stir and cook for 4 minutes.

2. Add zucchinis, salt and pepper, stir and cook for 4 minutes more.
3. Add pork, garlic powder, basil, more salt and pepper, stir and cook until meat is done.
4. Add mustard, stir, cook for 3 minutes more, divide into bowls and serve.

Enjoy!

Nutrition: calories 240, fat 15, fiber 2, carbs 9, protein 17

LUNCH: PESTO CHICKEN SALAD

The combination is absolutely delicious! You should try it!

Preparation time: 10 minutes

Cooking time: 0 minutes

Servings: 4

Ingredients:

- 1-pound chicken meat, cooked and cubed
- Salt and black pepper to the taste
- 10 cherry tomatoes, halved
- 6 bacon slices, cooked and crumbled
- ¼ cup mayonnaise
- 1 avocado, pitted, peeled and cubed
- 2 tablespoons garlic pesto

Directions:

1. In a salad bowl, mix chicken with bacon, avocado, tomatoes, salt and pepper and stir.
2. Add mayo and garlic pesto, toss well to coat and serve.

Enjoy!

Nutrition: calories 357, fat 23, fiber 5, carbs 3, protein 26

DINNER: LEMON CHICKEN

You'll soon see how easy this keto recipe is!

Preparation time: 10 minutes

Cooking time: 45 minutes

Servings: 6

Ingredients:

- 1 whole chicken, cut into medium pieces
- Salt and black pepper to the taste
- Juice from 2 lemons
- Zest from 2 lemons
- Lemon rinds from 2 lemons

Directions:

1. Put chicken pieces in a baking dish, season with salt and pepper to the taste and drizzle lemon juice.
2. Toss to coat well, add lemon zest and lemon rinds, introduce in the oven at 375 degrees F and bake for 45 minutes.
3. Discard lemon rinds, divide chicken between plates, drizzle sauce from the baking dish over it and serve.

Enjoy!

Nutrition: calories 334, fat 24, fiber 2, carbs 4.5, protein 27

DESSERT: LEMON MOUSSE

This is so refreshing and delicious!

Preparation time: 10 minutes

Cooking time: 0 minutes

Servings: 5

Ingredients:

- 1 cup heavy cream
- A pinch of salt
- 1 teaspoon lemon stevia
- ¼ cup lemon juice
- 8 ounces mascarpone cheese

Directions:

1. In a bowl, mix heavy cream with mascarpone and lemon juice and stir using your mixer.
2. Add a pinch of salt and stevia and blend everything.
3. Divide into dessert glasses and keep in the fridge until you serve.

Enjoy!

Nutrition: calories 265, fat 27, fiber 0, carbs 2, protein 4

DAY15

BREAKFAST: CASSEROLE

You've got to try this!

Preparation time: 10 minutes

Cooking time: 40 minutes

Servings: 4

Ingredients:

- 10 eggs
- 1-pound pork sausage, chopped
- 1 yellow onion, chopped
- 3 cups spinach, torn
- Salt and black pepper to the taste
- 3 tablespoons avocado oil

Directions:

1. Heat up a pan with 1 tablespoon oil over medium heat, add sausage, stir and brown it for 4 minutes.
2. Add onion, stir and cook for 3 minutes more.
3. Add spinach, stir and cook for 1 minute.
4. Grease a baking dish with the rest of the oil and spread sausage mix.
5. Whisk eggs and add them to sausage mix.

6. Stir gently, introduce in the oven at 350 degrees F and bake for 30 minutes.
7. Leave casserole to cool down for a few minutes before serving it for breakfast.

Enjoy!

Nutrition: calories 345, fat 12, fiber 1, carbs 8, protein 22

LUNCH: CRAB CAKES

Try these crab cakes for lunch! You won't regret it!

Preparation time: 10 minutes

Cooking time: 12 minutes

Servings: 6

Ingredients:

- 1-pound crabmeat
- ¼ cup parsley, chopped
- Salt and black pepper to the taste
- 2 green onions, chopped
- ¼ cup cilantro, chopped
- 1 teaspoon jalapeno pepper, minced
- 1 teaspoon lemon juice
- 1 teaspoon Worcestershire sauce
- 1 teaspoon old bay seasoning
- ½ teaspoon mustard powder
- ½ cup mayonnaise
- 1 egg
- 2 tablespoons olive oil

Directions:

1. In a large bowl mix crab meat with salt, pepper, parsley, green onions, cilantro, jalapeno, lemon

juice, old bay seasoning, mustard powder and Worcestershire sauce and stir very well.
2. In another bowl mix egg wit mayo and whisk.
3. Add this to crabmeat mix and stir everything.
4. Shape 6 patties from this mix and place them on a plate.
5. Heat up a pan with the oil over medium high heat, add 3 crab cakes, cook for 3 minutes, flip, cook them for 3 minutes more and transfer to paper towels.
6. Repeat with the other 3 crab cakes, drain excess grease and serve for lunch.

Enjoy!

Nutrition: calories 254, fat 17, fiber 1, carbs 1, protein 20

DINNER: SALMON WITH CAPER SAUCE

This dish is wonderful and very simple to make!

Preparation time: 10 minutes

Cooking time: 20 minutes

Servings: 3

Ingredients:

- 3 salmon fillets
- Salt and black pepper to the taste
- 1 tablespoon olive oil
- 1 tablespoon Italian seasoning
- 2 tablespoons capers
- 3 tablespoons lemon juice
- 4 garlic cloves, minced
- 2 tablespoons ghee

Directions:

1. Heat up a pan with the olive oil over medium heat, add fish fillets skin side up, season them with salt, pepper and Italian seasoning, cook for 2 minutes, flip and cook for 2 more minutes, take off heat, cover pan and leave aside for 15 minutes.
2. Transfer fish to a plate and leave them aside.

3. Heat up the same pan over medium heat, add capers, lemon juice and garlic, stir and cook for 2 minutes.
4. Take the pan off the heat, add ghee and stir very well.
5. Return fish to pan and toss to coat with the sauce.
6. Divide between plates and serve.

Enjoy!

Nutrition: calories 245, fat 12, fiber 1, carbs 3, protein 23

DESSERT: VANILLA ICE CREAM

Try this keto ice cream on a summer day!

Preparation time: 3 hours and 10 minutes

Cooking time: 0 minutes

Servings: 6

Ingredients:

- 4 eggs, yolks and whites separated
- ¼ teaspoon cream of tartar
- ½ cup swerve
- 1 tablespoon vanilla extract
- 1 and ¼ cup heavy whipping cream

Directions:

1. In a bowl, mix egg whites with cream of tartar and swerve and stir using your mixer.
2. In another bowl, whisk cream with vanilla extract and blend very well.
3. Combine the 2 mixtures and stir gently.
4. In another bowl, whisk egg yolks very well and then add the two egg whites mix.
5. Stir gently, pour this into a container and keep in the freezer for 3 hours before serving your ice cream.

Enjoy!

Nutrition: calories 243, fat 22, fiber 0, carbs 2, protein 4

DAY 16

BREAKFAST: PATTIES

This is incredibly tasty and easy to make for breakfast!

Preparation time: 10 minutes

Cooking time: 10 minutes

Servings: 4

Ingredients:

- 1-pound pork meat, minced
- Salt and black pepper to the taste
- ¼ teaspoon thyme, dried
- ½ teaspoon sage, dried
- ¼ teaspoon ginger, dried
- 3 tablespoon cold water
- 1 tablespoon coconut oil

Directions:

1. Put meat in a bowl.
2. In another bowl, mix water with salt, pepper, sage, thyme and ginger and whisk well.
3. Add this to meat and stir very well.

4. Shape your patties and place them on a working surface.
5. Heat up a pan with the coconut oil over medium high heat, add patties, fry them for 5 minutes, flip and cook them for 3 minutes more.
6. Serve them warm.

Enjoy!

Nutrition: calories 320, fat 13, fiber 2, carbs 10, protein 12

LUNCH: MUFFINS

These muffins will really get to your soul!

Preparation time: 10 minutes

Cooking time: 45 minutes

Servings: 13

Ingredients:

- 6 egg yolks
- 2 tablespoons coconut aminos
- ½ pound mushrooms
- ¾ cup coconut flour
- 1-pound beef, ground
- Salt to the taste

Directions:

1. In your food processor, mix mushrooms with salt, coconut aminos and egg yolks and blend well.
2. In a bowl, mix beef meat with some salt and stir.
3. Add mushroom mix to beef and stir everything.
4. Add coconut flour and stir again.

5. Divide this into 13 cupcake cups, introduce in the oven at 350 degrees f and bake for 45 minutes.
6. Serve them for lunch!

Enjoy!

Nutrition: calories 160, fat 10, fiber 3, carbs 1, protein 12

DINNER: FRIED CHICKEN AND PAPRIKA SAUCE

It's very healthy and it will make a great dinner idea!

Preparation time: 10 minutes

Cooking time: 20 minutes

Servings: 5

Ingredients:

- 1 tablespoon coconut oil
- 3 and ½ pounds chicken breasts
- 1 cup chicken stock
- 1 and ¼ cups yellow onion, chopped
- 1 tablespoon lime juice
- ¼ cup coconut milk
- 2 teaspoons paprika
- 1 teaspoon red pepper flakes
- 2 tablespoons green onions, chopped
- Salt and black pepper to the taste

Directions:

1. Heat up a pan with the oil over medium high heat, add chicken, cook for 2 minutes on each side, transfer to a plate and leave aside.

2. Reduce heat to medium, add onions to the pan and cook for 4 minutes.
3. Add stock, coconut milk, pepper flakes, paprika, lime juice, salt and pepper and stir well.
4. Return chicken to the pan, add more salt and pepper, cover pan and cook for 15 minutes.
5. Divide between plates and serve.

Enjoy!

Nutrition: calories 140, fat 4, fiber 3, carbs 3, protein 6

DESSERT: CHEESECAKE SQUARES

They look so good!

Preparation time: 10 minutes

Cooking time: 20 minutes

Servings: 9

Ingredients:

- 5 ounces coconut oil, melted
- ½ teaspoon baking powder
- 4 tablespoons swerve
- 1 teaspoon vanilla
- 4 ounces cream cheese
- 6 eggs
- ½ cup blueberries

Directions:

1. In a bowl, mix coconut oil with eggs, cream cheese, vanilla, swerve and baking powder and blend using an immersion blender.
2. Fold blueberries, pour everything into a square baking dish, introduce in the oven at 320 degrees F and bake for 20 minutes.

3. Leave you cake to cool down, slice into squares and serve.

Enjoy!

Nutrition: calories 220, fat 2, fiber 0.5, carbs 2, protein 4

DAY17

BREAKFAST: SAUSAGE QUICHE

It's so amazing! You must make it for breakfast tomorrow!

Preparation time: 10 minutes

Cooking time: 40 minutes

Servings: 6

Ingredients:

- 12 ounces pork sausage, chopped
- Salt and black pepper to the taste
- 2 teaspoons whipping cream
- 2 tablespoons parsley, chopped
- 10 mixed cherry tomatoes, halved
- 6 eggs
- 2 tablespoons parmesan, grated
- 5 eggplant slices

Directions:

1. Spread sausage pieces on the bottom of a baking dish.

2. Layer eggplant slices on top.
3. Add cherry tomatoes.
4. In a bowl, mix eggs with salt, pepper, cream and parmesan and whisk well.
5. Pour this into the baking dish, introduce in the oven at 375 degrees F and bake for 40 minutes.
6. Serve right away.

Enjoy!

Nutrition: calories 340, fat 28, fiber 3, carbs 3, protein 17

LUNCH: PORK PIE

This is something you've been craving for a very long time! Don't worry! It's a keto idea!

Preparation time: 10 minutes

Cooking time: 50 minutes

Servings: 6

Ingredients:

For the pie crust:

- 2 cups cracklings
- ¼ cup flax meal
- 1 cup almond flour
- 2 eggs
- A pinch of salt

For the filling:

- 1 cup cheddar cheese, grated
- 4 eggs
- 12 ounces pork loin, chopped
- 6 bacon slices
- ½ cup cream cheese
- 1 red onion, chopped

- ¼ cup chives, chopped
- 2 garlic cloves, minced
- Salt and black pepper to the taste
- 2 tablespoons ghee

Directions:

1. In your food processor, mix cracklings with almond flour, flax meal, 2 eggs and salt and blend until you obtain a dough.
2. Transfer this to a pie pan and press well on the bottom.
3. Introduce in the oven at 350 degrees F and bake for 15 minutes.
4. Meanwhile, heat up a pan with the ghee over medium high heat, add garlic and onion, stir and cook for 5 minutes.
5. Add bacon, stir and cook for 5 minutes.
6. Add pork loin, cook until it's brown on all sides and take off heat.
7. In a bowl, mix eggs with salt, pepper, cheddar cheese and cream cheese and blend well.
8. Add chives and stir again.
9. Spread pork into pie pan, add eggs mix, introduce in the oven at 350 degrees F and bake for 25 minutes.
10. Leave the pie to cool down for a couple of minutes and serve.

Enjoy!

Nutrition: calories 455, fat 34, fiber 3, carbs 3, protein 33

DINNER: GRILLED OYSTERS

These are so juicy and delicious!

Preparation time: 10 minutes

Cooking time: 10 minutes

Servings: 3

Ingredients:

- 6 big oysters, shucked
- 3 garlic cloves, minced
- 1 lemon cut in wedges
- 1 tablespoon parsley
- A pinch of sweet paprika
- 2 tablespoons melted ghee

Directions:

1. Top each oyster with melted ghee, parsley, paprika and ghee.
2. Place them on preheated grill over medium high heat and cook for 8 minutes.
3. Serve them with lemon wedges on the side.

Enjoy!

Nutrition: calories 60, fat 1, fiber 0, carbs 0.6, protein 1

DESSERT: TASTY BROWNIES

These flourless keto brownies are excellent!

Preparation time: 10 minutes

Cooking time: 20 minutes

Servings: 12

Ingredients:

- 6 ounces coconut oil, melted
- 6 eggs
- 3 ounces cocoa powder
- 2 teaspoons vanilla
- ½ teaspoon baking powder
- 4 ounces cream cheese
- 5 tablespoons swerve

Directions:

1. In a blender, mix eggs with coconut oil, cocoa powder, baking powder, vanilla, cream cheese and swerve and stir using a mixer.
2. Pour this into a lined baking dish, introduce in the oven at 350 degrees F and bake for 20 minutes.
3. Slice into rectangle pieces when their cold and serve.

Enjoy!

Nutrition: calories 178, fat 14, fiber 2, carbs 3, protein 5

DAY18

BREAKFAST JOY

This is a Ketogenic breakfast worth trying!

Preparation time: 10 minutes

Cooking time: 40 minutes

Servings: 6

Ingredients:

- 1 pound sausage, chopped
- 1 leek, chopped
- 8 eggs, whisked
- ¼ cup coconut milk
- 6 asparagus stalks, chopped
- 1 tablespoon dill, chopped
- Salt and black pepper to the taste
- ¼ teaspoon garlic powder
- 1 tablespoon coconut oil, melted

Directions:

1. Heat up a pan over medium heat, add sausage pieces and brown them for a few minutes.

2. Add asparagus and leek, stir and cook for a few minutes.
3. Meanwhile, in a bowl, mix eggs with salt, pepper, dill, garlic powder and coconut milk and whisk well.
4. Pour this into a baking dish which you've greased with the coconut oil.
5. Add sausage and veggies on top and whisk everything.
6. Introduce in the oven at 325 degrees F and bake for 40 minutes.
7. Serve warm.

Enjoy!

Nutrition: calories 340, fat 12, fiber 3, carbs 8, protein 23

LUNCH: PATE

Enjoy something really easy to launch: a Ketogenic liver pate!

Preparation time: 10 minutes

Cooking time: 0 minutes

Servings: 1

Ingredients:

- 4 ounces chicken livers, sautéed
- 1 teaspoon mixed thyme, sage and oregano, chopped
- Salt and black pepper to the taste
- 3 tablespoons butter
- 3 radishes, thinly sliced
- Crusted bread slices for serving

Directions:

- In your food processor, mix chicken livers with thyme, sage, oregano, butter, salt and pepper and blend very well for a few minutes.
- Spread on crusted bread slices and top with radishes slices.
- Serve right away.

Enjoy!

Nutrition: calories 380, fat 40, fiber 5, carbs 1, protein 17

DINNER: CHICKEN FAJITAS

Are you in the mood for some tasty Mexican style food? Then, try this next idea!

Preparation time: 10 minutes

Cooking time: 15 minutes

Servings: 4

Ingredients:

- 2 pounds chicken breasts, skinless, boneless and cut into strips
- 1 teaspoon garlic powder
- 1 teaspoon chili powder
- 2 teaspoons cumin
- 2 tablespoons lime juice
- Salt and black pepper to the taste
- 1 teaspoon sweet paprika
- 2 tablespoons coconut oil
- 1 teaspoon coriander, ground
- 1 green bell pepper, sliced
- 1 red bell pepper, sliced
- 1 yellow onion, sliced
- 1 tablespoon cilantro, chopped
- 1 avocado, pitted, peeled and sliced
- 2 limes, cut into wedges

Directions:

1. In a bowl, mix lime juice with chili powder, cumin, salt, pepper, garlic powder, paprika and coriander and stir.
2. Add chicken pieces and toss to coat well.
3. Heat up a pan with half of the oil over medium high heat, add chicken, cook for 3 minutes on each side and transfer to a bowl.
4. Heat up the pan with the rest of the oil over medium heat, add onion and all bell peppers, stir and cook for 6 minutes.
5. Return chicken to pan, add more salt and pepper, stir and divide between plates.
6. Top with avocado, lime wedges and cilantro and serve.

Enjoy!

Nutrition: calories 240, fat 10, fiber 2, carbs 5, protein 20

DESSERT: CHOCOLATE PUDDING

This pudding is so tasty!

Preparation time: 50 minutes

Cooking time: 5 minutes

Servings: 2

Ingredients:

- 2 tablespoons water
- 1 tablespoon gelatin
- 2 tablespoons maple syrup
- ½ teaspoon stevia powder
- 2 tablespoons cocoa powder
- 1 cup coconut milk

Directions:

1. Heat up a pan with the coconut milk over medium heat, add stevia and cocoa powder and stir well.
2. In a bowl, mix gelatin with water, stir well and add to the pan.
3. Stir well, add maple syrup, whisk again, divide into ramekins and keep in the fridge for 45 minutes.

4. Serve cold.

Enjoy!

Nutrition: calories 140, fat 2, fiber 2, carbs 4, protein 4

DAY19

BREAKFAST: CHORIZO & CAULIFLOWER

You don't need to be an expert cook to make a great breakfast! Try this next recipe and enjoy!

Preparation time: 10 minutes

Cooking time: 45 minutes

Servings: 4

Ingredients:

- 1-pound chorizo, chopped
- 12 ounces canned green chilies, chopped
- 1 yellow onion, chopped
- ½ teaspoon garlic powder
- Salt and black pepper to the taste
- 1 cauliflower head, florets separated
- 4 eggs, whisked
- 2 tablespoons green onions, chopped

Directions:

1. Heat up a pan over medium heat, add chorizo and onion, stir and brown for a few minutes.

2. Add green chilies, stir, cook for a few minutes and take off heat.
3. In your food processor mix cauliflower with some salt and pepper and blend.
4. Transfer this to a bowl, add eggs, salt, pepper and garlic powder and whisk everything.
5. Add chorizo mix as well, whisk again and transfer everything to a greased baking dish.
6. Bake in the oven at 375 degrees F and bake for 40 minutes.
7. Leave casserole to cool down for a few minutes, sprinkle green onions on top, slice and serve.

Enjoy!

Nutrition: calories 350, fat 12, fiber 4, carbs 6, protein 20

LUNCH: CHOWDER

You might end up adoring this chowder! Try it at least once!

Preparation time: 10 minutes

Cooking time: 4 hours

Servings: 4

Ingredients:

- 1-pound chicken thighs, skinless and boneless
- 10 ounces canned tomatoes, chopped
- 1 cup chicken stock
- 8 ounces cream cheese
- Juice from 1 lime
- Salt and black pepper to the taste
- 1 jalapeno pepper, chopped
- 1 yellow onion, chopped
- 2 tablespoons cilantro, chopped
- 1 garlic clove, minced
- Cheddar cheese, shredded for serving
- Lime wedges for serving

Directions:

1. In your crock pot, mix chicken with tomatoes, stock, cream cheese, salt, pepper, lime juice, jalapeno, onion, garlic and cilantro, stir, cover and cook on High for 4 hours.
2. Uncover pot, shred meat into the pot, divide into bowls and serve with cheddar cheese on top and lime wedges on the side.

Enjoy!

Nutrition: calories 300, fat 5, fiber 6, carbs 3, protein 26

DINNER: BAKED HALIBUT

This is a delicious fish and if you choose to make it this way you will really end up loving it!

Preparation time: 10 minutes

Cooking time: 10 minutes

Servings: 4

Ingredients:

- ½ cup parmesan, grated
- ¼ cup ghee
- ¼ cup mayonnaise
- 2 tablespoons green onions, chopped
- 6 garlic cloves, minced
- A dash of Tabasco sauce
- 4 halibut fillets
- Salt and black pepper to the taste
- Juice of ½ lemon

Directions:

1. Season halibut with salt, pepper and some of the lemon juice, place in a baking dish and cook in the oven at 450 degrees F for 6 minutes.

2. Meanwhile, heat up a pan with the ghee over medium heat, add parmesan, mayo, green onions, Tabasco sauce, garlic and the rest of the lemon juice and stir well.
3. Take fish out of the oven, drizzle parmesan sauce all over, turn oven to broil and broil your fish for 3 minutes.
4. Divide between plates and serve.

Enjoy!

Nutrition: calories 240, fat 12, fiber 1, carbs 5, protein 23

DESSERT: SIMPLE AVOCADO PUDDING

This is so easy to make at home and it follows keto principles!

Preparation time: 10 minutes

Cooking time: 0 minutes

Servings: 4

Ingredients:

- 2 avocados, pitted, peeled and chopped
- 2 teaspoons vanilla extract
- 80 drops stevia
- 1 tablespoon lime juice
- 14 ounces canned coconut milk

Directions:

1. In your blender, mix avocado with coconut milk, vanilla extract, stevia and lime juice, blend well, spoon into dessert bowls and keep in the fridge until you serve it.

Enjoy!

Nutrition: calories 150, fat 3, fiber 3, carbs 5, protein 6

DAY20

BREAKFAST: ITALIAN SPAGHETTI CASSEROLE

Try an Italian Ketogenic breakfast today!

Preparation time: 10 minutes

Cooking time: 55 minutes

Servings: 4

Ingredients:

- 4 tablespoons ghee
- 1 squash, halved
- Salt and black pepper to the taste
- ½ cup tomatoes, chopped
- 2 garlic cloves, minced
- 1 cup yellow onion, chopped
- ½ teaspoon Italian seasoning
- 3 ounces Italian salami, chopped
- ½ cup kalamata olives, chopped
- 4 eggs
- A handful parsley, chopped

Directions:

1. Place squash halves on a lined baking sheet, season with salt and pepper, spread 1 tablespoon ghee over them, introduce in the oven at 400 degrees F and bake for 45 minutes.
2. Meanwhile, heat up a pan with the rest of the ghee over medium heat, add garlic, onions, salt and pepper, stir and cook for a couple of minutes.
3. Add salami and tomatoes, stir and cook for 10 minutes.
4. Add olives, stir and cook for a few minutes more.
5. Take squash halves out of the oven, scrape flesh with a fork and add over salami mix into the pan.
6. Stir, make 4 holes in the mix, crack an egg in each, season with salt and pepper, introduce pan in the oven at 400 degrees F and bake until eggs are done.
7. Sprinkle parsley on top and serve.

Enjoy!

Nutrition: calories 333, fat 23, fiber 4, carbs 12, protein 15

LUNCH: COCONUT SOUP

Try this Ketogenic coconut soup really soon! Everyone will love it!

Preparation time: 10 minutes

Cooking time: 30 minutes

Servings: 2

Ingredients:

- 4 cups chicken stock
- 3 lime leaves
- 1 and ½ cups coconut milk
- 1 teaspoon lemongrass, dried
- 1 cup cilantro, chopped
- 1-inch ginger, grated
- 4 Thai chilies, dried and chopped
- Salt and black pepper to the taste
- 4 ounces shrimp, raw, peeled and deveined
- 2 tablespoons red onion, chopped
- 1 tablespoon coconut oil
- 2 tablespoons mushrooms, chopped
- 1 tablespoon fish sauce
- 1 tablespoon cilantro, chopped
- Juice from 1 lime

Directions:

1. In a pot, mix chicken stock with coconut milk, lime leaves, lemongrass, Thai chilies, 1 cup cilantro, ginger, salt and pepper, stir, bring to a simmer over medium heat, cook for 20 minutes, strain and return to pot.
2. Heat up soup again over medium heat, add coconut oil, shrimp, fish sauce, mushrooms and onions, stir and cook for 10 minutes more.
3. Add lime juice and 1 tablespoon cilantro, stir, ladle into bowls and serve for lunch!

Enjoy!

Nutrition: calories 450, fat 34, fiber 4, carbs 8, protein 12

DINNER: SKILLET CHICKEN WITH MUSHROOMS

The combination is absolutely delicious! We guarantee it!

Preparation time: 10 minutes

Cooking time: 30 minutes

Servings: 4

Ingredients:

- 4 chicken thighs
- 2 cups mushrooms, sliced
- ¼ cup ghee
- Salt and black pepper to the taste
- ½ teaspoon onion powder
- ½ teaspoon garlic powder
- ½ cup water
- 1 teaspoon Dijon mustard
- 1 tablespoon tarragon, chopped

Directions:

1. Heat up a pan with half of the ghee over medium high heat, add chicken thighs, season them with salt, pepper, garlic powder and onion powder, cook the for 3 minutes on each side and transfer to a bowl.

2. Heat up the same pan with the rest of the ghee over medium high heat, add mushrooms, stir and cook for 5 minutes.
3. Add mustard and water and stir well.
4. Return chicken pieces to the pan, stir, cover and cook for 15 minutes.
5. Add tarragon, stir, cook for 5 minutes, divide between plates and serve.

Enjoy!

Nutrition: calories 453, fat 32, fiber 6, carbs 1, protein 36

DESSERT: MINT DELIGHT

It has such a fresh texture and taste!

Preparation time: 2 hours and 10 minutes

Cooking time: 0 minutes

Servings: 3

Ingredients:

- ½ cup coconut oil, melted
- 3 stevia drops
- 1 tablespoon cocoa powder

For the pudding:

- 1 teaspoon peppermint oil
- 14 ounces canned coconut milk
- 1 avocado, pitted, peeled and chopped
- 10 drops stevia

Directions:

1. In a bowl, mix coconut oil with cocoa powder and 3 drops stevia, stir well, transfer to a lined container and keep in the fridge for 1 hour.
2. Chop this into small pieces and leave aside for now.

3. In your blender, mix coconut milk with avocado, 10 drops stevia and peppermint oil and pulse well.
4. Add chocolate chips, fold them gently, divide pudding into bowls and keep in the fridge for 1 more hour.

Enjoy!

Nutrition: calories 140, fat 3, fiber 2, carbs 3, protein 4

DAY21

BREAKFAST PORRIDGE

This is just delicious!

Preparation time: 5 minutes

Cooking time: 10 minutes

Servings: 1

Ingredients:

- 1 teaspoon cinnamon powder
- A pinch of nutmeg
- ½ cup almonds, ground
- 1 teaspoon stevia
- ¾ cup coconut cream
- A pinch of cardamom, ground
- A pinch of cloves, ground

Directions:

1. Heat up a pan over medium heat, add coconut cream and heat up for a few minutes.
2. Add stevia and almonds and stir well for 5 minutes.
3. Add cloves, cardamom, nutmeg and cinnamon and stir well.

4. Transfer to a bowl and serve hot.

Enjoy!

Nutrition: calories 200, fat 12, fiber 4, carbs 8, protein 16

LUNCH: ZUCCHINI NOODLES SOUP

This Ketogenic soup is simple and very tasty!

Preparation time: 10 minutes

Cooking time: 15 minutes

Servings: 8

Ingredients:

- 1 small yellow onion, chopped
- 2 garlic cloves, minced
- 1 jalapeno pepper, chopped
- 1 tablespoon coconut oil
- 1 and ½ tablespoons curry paste
- 6 cups chicken stock
- 15 ounces canned coconut milk
- 1-pound chicken breasts, sliced
- 1 red bell pepper, sliced
- 2 tablespoons fish sauce
- 2 zucchinis, cut with a spiralizer
- ½ cup cilantro, chopped
- Lime wedges for serving

Directions:

1. Heat up a pot with the oil over medium heat, add onion, stir and cook for 5 minutes.

2. Add garlic, jalapeno and curry paste, stir and cook for 1 minute.
3. Add stock and coconut milk, stir and bring to a boil.
4. Add red bell pepper, chicken and fish sauce, stir and simmer for 4 minutes more.
5. Add cilantro, stir, cook for 1 minute and take off heat.
6. Divide zucchini noodles into soup bowls, add soup on top and serve with lime wedges on the side.

Enjoy!

Nutrition: calories 287, fat 14, fiber 2, carbs 7, protein 25

DINNER: CRUSTED SALMON

The crust is wonderful!

Preparation time: 10 minutes

Cooking time: 15 minutes

Servings: 4

Ingredients:

- 3 garlic cloves, minced
- 2 pounds salmon fillet
- Salt and black pepper to the taste
- ½ cup parmesan, grated
- ¼ cup parsley, chopped

Directions:

1. Place salmon on a lined baking sheet, season with salt and pepper, cover with a parchment paper, introduce in the oven at 425 degrees F and bake for 10 minutes.
2. Take fish out of the oven, sprinkle parmesan, parsley and garlic over fish, introduce in the oven again and cook for 5 minutes more.
3. Divide between plates and serve.

Enjoy!

Nutrition: calories 240, fat 12, fiber 1, carbs 0.6, protein 25

DESSERT: AMAZING COCONUT PUDDING

You've got to love this keto pudding!

Preparation time: 10 minutes

Cooking time: 10 minutes

Servings: 4

Ingredients:

- 1 and 2/3 cups coconut milk
- 1 tablespoon gelatin
- 6 tablespoons swerve
- 3 egg yolks
- ½ teaspoon vanilla extract

Directions:

1. In a bowl, mix gelatin with 1 tablespoon coconut milk, stir well and leave aside for now.
2. Put the rest of the milk into a pan and heat up over medium heat.
3. Add swerve, stir and cook for 5 minutes.
4. In a bowl, mix egg yolks with the hot coconut milk and vanilla extract, stir well and return everything to the pan.
5. Cook for 4 minutes, add gelatin and stir well.

6. Divide this into 4 ramekins and keep your pudding in the fridge until you serve it.

Enjoy!

Nutrition: calories 140, fat 2, fiber 0, carbs 2, protein 2

FAQS

What is a ketone?

A ketone is a side-effect of fat being burned. It is fundamentally an elective source of vitality (fuel) from glucose. Ketones are the favored fuel for the body and progressively effective for the mind and the heart.

I began the keto diet about seven days prior. Presently I'm drained always. What do I do?

As your body acclimates to fat consuming, you will require more B vitamins. The supplement you need a ton of to fend off the tiredness and help your adrenals and digestion is B5. A sodium deficiency could likewise create tiredness and weakness.

How might I maintain a strategic distance from (or get over) the keto influenza?

The side effects of keto influenza are migraines, body throbs, cravings, mind mist, and weariness. Simply consider what you're endeavoring to do. You're changing over your entire cell apparatus to fat consuming. What you have to do to maintain a strategic distance from or recuperate the keto influenza is get more electrolytes and B vitamins.

These are the cofactors that assist in building up the apparatus to consume fat viably without depleting your body. For the B vitamins, try nutritional yeast. Nonetheless, nutritional yeast does not have B5 so you may need to take a B5 supplement. I prescribe electrolyte powder.

It has 1,000 mgs of potassium and will enable you to get to 4,700 mgs you need to make this apparatus to consume fat quicker and get into ketosis!

Will excessively protein toss me out of ketosis?

Yes, particularly an excessive amount of lean protein—like turkey and chicken and even lean fish. Egg white without the yolk is lean protein and will trigger insulin more than the whole egg. Regularly three to six ounces of protein is adequate, and 10+ ounces is going to kick you out of ketosis.

How long before I begin shedding pounds?

A lot of times, individuals need this to begin happening immediately. Your body has been running on glucose for as long as you can remember, however. Your cells need to fabricate new enzymes an entirely different cell machine, to breakdown fat as another wellspring of fuel. It might occur in a month, however almost certain, it will take something like a month and a half. Be that as it may, when you do arrive you won't have sugar yearnings any longer. You'll have better glucose. Your memory will be more improved and you'll urinate less around evening time and rest better on the grounds that your blood sugar won't dive during the night after sugar spikes.

Alright, I "tumbled off the wagon" and cheated. To what extent will it take me to get once more into ketosis now?

It can take 48– 72 hours in case you're fortunate, yet it could be as long as seven days. Presently, in case you're in your twenties and truly healthy, you'll bounce back in a day. When you're more established and taking a shot at fixing a broken metabolism, it will take longer.

Will vegetables moderate ketosis?

The appropriate response is no. For whatever length of time that you keep away from vegetables like corn, beets, and carrots, which are high in starch and sugar (particularly carrot JUICE, which is stuffed with sugar), you don't need to stress over the vegetable family.

Indeed, you need to eat loads of green verdant vegetables, cruciferous vegetables and Brussel sprouts. Make huge kale plates of salads with bacon bits and a full-fat dressing. Or on the other hand make beet greens sautéed in coconut oil with some bacon, garlic, and onion blended in. These will be dishes packed with potassium, which will calm food desires much like fat does. Frequently, food desires are just your body shouting out for minerals and nutrients you're not giving it.

Would it be a good idea for me to count total carbs or net carbs?

Check net carbs, which is all out carbs excluding fiber.

Is it conceivable to eat excessive fat?

Yes. In the event that you look into the keto diet on the web, they state to consume 85% of calories from fat. On the off chance that you devour 2500 calories from fat, you are consuming 220 grams of fat for each day. I trust this is excessive and could forestall fat burning in light of the fact that at that point you'd kept running on the fat you're consuming as opposed to your fat stores. First and foremost, you'll require progressive fat to go starting with one meal then onto the next; in any case, as you completely adjust, you'll need less in light of the fact that you'll keep running on your own body fat.

What amount of fat would it be advisable for me to eat every meal?

In case you're truly doing combating a high hunger/high craving day or week, you should need to include more fat, particularly at breakfast to trim your hunger for the duration of the day and empower you to go longer without longings and craving.

Ketosis when all is said and done suppresses your craving, so your yearning will be extraordinarily decreased. You will probably go numerous hours without eating. Give the yearning a chance to manage how much fat you eat. In case you're not hungry, cut down on the fat a tad.

Virginia Cooke

KETOGENIC DIET FOR WOMEN

The Complete 2020 Guide to Lose Weight Quickly, Heal Your Body and Reset Your Metabolism With 14-days Meal Plan and 100+ Delicious Recipes and Steps

VIRGINIA COOKE

PREFACE

The ketogenic diet or a keto diet is a proposed diet or meal plan which is low or deficient in carbohydrate level, meaning; is a low-carb, high-fat diet plan recommended by the dietician or a physician that offers many health benefits.

As part of the effort to maintain steady health status, ketogenic diet offers and as well can help to lose excessive body weight and improve general health. The ketogenic diet also offers benefits like the treatment of cancer, treatment of epilepsy and the treatment of Alzheimer's.

Most women these days suffer from different sorts of diseases and health challenges due to intake of carbohydrate. The reduction in carbohydrates makes the body to be metabolic a state called Ketosis. Then, the body becomes vast in burning fats and convert it into energy.

Likewise, it turns fats into ketones, especially in the liver, which then supply energy for the brain.

The ketogenic diet can cause drastic reductions in the insulin levels, the blood sugar. There are lots of benefits women derive from the ketogenic diets such as regulation in hormonal level, control in the menstrual cycle and much more.

This book offers women so many benefits for a variety of health conditions such as;

- Hearth diseases

- Cancer
- Brain injuries
- Alzheimer's diseases
- Epilepsy
- Polycystic ovary syndrome
- Acne
- Parkinson's diseases and lots more.

CHAPTER 1: GENERAL UNDERSTANDING OF KETOGENIC DIET

What is ketosis?

Ketosis is a metabolic state wherein your body uses fat and ketones instead of glucose (sugar) as its primary fuel source.

Glucose is put away in your liver and discharged as required for vitality. Be that as it may, after carb admission has been incredibly low for one to two days, these glucose stores become exhausted. Your liver can make some glucose from amino acids in the protein you eat through a procedure known as gluconeogenesis, however not about enough to address the issues of your cerebrum, which requires a steady fuel supply.

Ketosis can supply you with an elective wellspring of energy.

In ketosis, your body produces ketones at a quickened rate. Ketones, or ketone bodies, are made by your liver from fat that you eat and your very own muscle versus fat. The three ketone bodies are Beta-Hydroxybutyrate (BHB), acetoacetate and CH3)2CO. (even though CH3)2CO is a breakdown result of acetoacetate).

Notwithstanding when on a higher-carb diet, your liver creates ketones all the time – principally medium-term while you rest – however generally just in small sums. In any case, when glucose and insulin levels decline on a carb-confined eating regimen, the liver increases its creation of ketones to give vitality to your cerebrum.

When the degree of ketones in your blood arrives at a specific limit, you are viewed as in healthy ketosis. Albeit both fasting and a keto diet will enable you to accomplish ketosis, just a keto diet is economical over significant lots of time. It has all the earmarks of being a reliable method to eat that can be pursued inconclusively.

Advantages of ketosis

Notwithstanding giving a reasonable vitality source, ketones – and specifically BHB – may help lessen aggravation and oxidative pressure. Which are accepted to assume a job in the improvement of numerous constant maladies?

There are a few setup advantages and potential advantages of being in wholesome ketosis.

Built-up advantages:

- Appetite recommendation: One of the primary things' individuals see when they're in ketosis is that they're never again hungry always. Examine has demonstrated that being in ketosis smothers craving.
- Weight loss: Most individuals naturally eat less when they confine carbs and are permitted as much fat and protein as they have to feel full. Since ketogenic diets smother craving, decline insulin levels, and increment fat consuming. It is-

n't unusual that they've been appeared to beat different eating regimens planned for weight reduction.
- Reversal of diabetes and prediabetes: In individuals with sort two diabetes or prediabetes. Being in ketosis can help standardize glucose and insulin reaction, prompting the stopping of diabetes drug.
- Potentially upgraded athletic execution: Ketosis may give a very enduring fuel supply during continued exercise in both abnormal state and recreational competitors.
- Seizure the board: Maintaining ketosis with the traditional ketogenic diet or less stringent adjusted Atkins diet (MAD) has been demonstrated compelling for controlling epilepsy in the two youngsters and grown-ups who don't react to hostile to seizure medicine.

What Is a Ketogenic Diet?

The ketogenic diet is an eating regimen that is a) high in fat and b) low in starches and proteins to constrain the body to depend on fat rather than sugars for vitality.

A ketogenic diet places the body in a condition of ketosis, where the essential fuel for the body is a separated result of fat called ketone bodies. Ketosis can happen through the decrease of sugars in the eating regimen or through fasting (or through taking an outer ketone-creating item). The liver produces ketone bodies by separating unsaturated fats, either from muscle to fat ratio or the fat that we eat.

This is rather than the body's fuel source when not in ketosis: sugars, which the body separates into glucose.

It is imperative to take note that there is a distinction between consuming dietary fat for fuel and getting the body to use put away fat.

The ketogenic diet is an extremely low-carbohydrate, high-fat eating routine that offers numerous similitudes with the Atkins and low-carb eats fewer carbs.

It includes radically lessening sugar admission and supplanting it with fat. This decrease in carbs places the body into a metabolic condition called the ketosis.

At the point when this happened, the body turns out to be unfathomably productive at consuming fat for vitality. It likewise converts fat into ketones in the liver, which can supply energy for the cerebrum.

Ketogenic diets can cause significant decreases in glucose and insulin intake in or levels. This, alongside the expanded ketones, has various medical advantages.

A regular low starch diet may mainly concentrate on restricting sugar with liberal measures of different sustenance's, without a particular accentuation on fats. It is anything but challenging to generally eat meats and some other non-starch nourishments for a low sugar diet, and not get into ketosis.

So, what's unique? The ketogenic diet goes above and beyond and limits protein too to accomplish ketosis. A ketogenic diet is contained:

- 65 – 80% of calories from fat

- 10 – 15% of calories from proteins (0.5 gram per lb of fit weight)
- 5 – 10% calories from starches.

Various Types of Ketogenic Diets

There are a few renditions of the ketogenic diet, including:

- The standard ketogenic diet (SKD): Ths a low-carb, moderate-protein, and high-fat diet. It regularly contains 75% fat, 20% protein, and just 5% carbs (1).
- The cyclical ketogenic diet (CKD): This diet includes times of higher-carb refeeds. For example, five ketogenic days pursued by two high-carb days.
- The targeted ketogenic diet (TKD): This diet enables you to include and target some diets carbs with exercises.
- High-protein ketogenic diet: This is like an example of a standard ketogenic diet, yet incorporates more protein. The proportion is regularly 60% fat, 35% protein, and 5% carbs.

Nonetheless, just the standard and high-protein ketogenic diets have been examined widely. Repetitive or focused on ketogenic diets are further developed strategies and utilized by muscle heads or competitors.

Other Health Benefits of Keto

The ketogenic diet started as a device for treating neurological illnesses, for example, epilepsy. Keto diet can have benefits for a wide range of wellbeing conditions:

- Heart infection: The ketogenic diet can improve hazard components like a muscle to fat ratio. HDL cholesterol levels, circulatory strain, and glucose.
- Cancer: The diet is at present, being utilized to treat a few types of malignant growth and moderate tumour development.
- Alzheimer's ailment: The keto diet may lessen side effects of Alzheimer's sickness and how to moderate its movement.
- Epilepsy: The ketogenic diet can cause large decreases in seizures in epileptic kids.
- Parkinson's ailment: One investigation found that the diet improved the side effects of Parkinson's illness.
- Polycystic ovary disorder: The ketogenic diet plan or routine can help decrease insulin levels, which may assume a vital job in polycystic ovary disorder.
- Brain wounds: One creature concentrate found that the diet can diminish blackouts and help recuperation after cerebrum damage.
- Acne: This lowers insulin levels and eating less sugar or handled sustenance may help improve skin break out.

Instructions to Eat Keto

In a perfect world, a keto diet ought to be gathered with whole and nutritious food that doesn't cause inflammation. This implies the 5-10% of the sugars would be from vegetables, nuts, and seeds as opposed to another wellspring of starch.

On a keto-type diet, the plate should comprise of for the most part non-bland vegetables, a sensible segment of meat (around 3 ounces), and a liberal measure of good fats. The fats can be nuts, seeds, olive oil, avocados, avocado oil, fed fat or bacon, grass-bolstered spread, MCT oil, or a topping like a sound mayo produced using these.

When an individual is keto-adjusted, the hunger is regularly directed. Instead of inclination denied, it is reasonable to feel less hungry in general and customarily slanted to abandon eating for 12 hours medium-term. This type of broadened fasting may give some additional medical advantages also.

Nourishments to Avoid

Any nourishment that is high in carbs ought to be restricted.

Here is a rundown of nourishments that should be diminished or wiped out on a ketogenic diet:

- Sugary nourishments: Soda, organic product juice, smoothies, cake, dessert, sweet, and so on
- Grains or starches: Wheat-based items, oat, pasta, rice, and so on.

- Fruit: All organic product, except for little parts of berries like strawberries.
- Beans or vegetables: Chickpeas, Peas, kidney beans, lentils, and so forth.
- Root vegetables and tubers: carrot, sweet potatoes, Potatoes, parsnips, and so forth.
- Low-fat or diet items: These are exceptionally handled and regularly high in carbs.
- Some fixings or sauces: These frequently contain sugar and undesirable fat.
- Unhealthy fats: Limit your admission of prepared vegetable oils, mayonnaise, and so on.
- Alcohol: Due to their high carb content, numerous mixed refreshments can toss you out of ketosis.
- Sugar diet sustenance's: These are frequently high in sugar alcohols, which can influence ketone levels sometimes. These foods likewise will, in general, be thoroughly handled.

Nourishments to Eat

You should base most of your suppers around this food:

- Meat: Red meat, chicken, steak, ham, sausage, bacon, and turkey.
- Fatty fish: Example such as salmon, trout, fish, and mackerel.
- Eggs: Look for fed or omega-3 entire eggs.
- Butter and cream: Look for grass-bolstered when conceivable.
- Cheese: Unprocessed (cheddar, goat, cream, blue, or mozzarella).

- Nuts and seeds: Examples like Almonds, pecans, flax seeds, pumpkin seeds, chia seeds, and so on.
- Healthy oils: Primarily additional virgin olive oil, and avocado oil.
- Avocados: Whole avocados or crisply made guacamole.
- Low-carb vegetable: Most onions, green vegetables, tomatoes, onions, peppers, and so on.
- Condiments: You can utilize pepper, salt, and different sound herbs and flavours.

It is ideal for putting together your diet for the most part concerning entire, single-fixing sustenance.

A KETOGENIC DIET FOR WOMEN

The Keto Diet, or Ketogenic Diet, is an eating regimen that is a) high in fat and b) low in starches and proteins to constrain the body to depend on fat rather than sugars for vitality for women.

This diet depends on a high consumption or intake of protein and fat, for example, meat, fish, olive oil, eggs, and limited quantities of vegetables. Ladies can encounter various medical advantages with this diet, including hormonal equalization, weight reduction, and even an enemy of maturing impact. You ought to meet your primary care physician before embraced this diet as it very well may be healthfully prohibitive. A multivitamin and mineral ought to be taken to enhance the Ketogenic Diet.

Types Of Keto Diet For Women

There basically three types of ketogenic diet plan for women. This type of ketogenic diet plan can be divided into three subgroups:

- Dirty Keto diet
- Lazy keto diet
- Exemplary keto diet

Exemplary Keto (additionally now called clean Keto) is essentially a method for eating where you limit your carbs and eat adequate protein and fat. Individuals who pursue great Keto will, in general track their macros utilizing an application or tracker or something to that effect. The ordinary macros for Keto are 5% carbs, 10-25% protein, and 65-85% fat.

Great clean Keto is related to utilizing fantastic fats, for example, olive oil, coconut oil and avocados, natural proteins where conceivable and excellent natural carbs, for example, greens. Individuals who eat clean Keto, for the most part, maintain a strategic distance from sugars and prepared nourishments, for example, keto bars and pre-packaged keto snacks.

Lazy Keto can mean a couple of various things. A few people don't follow their macros and maintain a strategic distance from carbs. Some will follow just carbs, holding them under 20 grams; for instance, however, they don't follow the rest.

Numerous individuals will begin with great Keto, get more fit, and continuously fall into an example of lazy Keto. This may work for support, yet if their weight begins to crawl up once more, they may need to return to clean Keto.

For individuals that begin with lazy Keto, they may lose some weight, and they will profit Healthwise yet. In the end, they will find that they have to 'tidy up' their Keto to proceed with weight reduction.

Dirty Keto is anything goes as long as they can fit it into their macros. The macros are equivalent to exemplary Keto, yet individuals who pursue dirty Keto don't stress such a significant amount over the nature of what they are eating as long as the sustenance accommodates their macros.

They will eat those instant keto bars and tidbits, discover things at their preferred cheap food spots to eat, and for the most part abstain from worrying about the fixings records on those jugs of sans sugar syrups.

Which Keto is better, exemplary, dirty, or lazy?

Even though there are upsides and downsides to every one of the three of these keto variants, none are terrible, and each of the three can fill a need for somebody who pursues Keto.

I feel that numerous individuals move around and cover between spotless, lazy and dirty Keto relying upon what's going on in their lives or even what sustenance may be accessible, state for instance during a get-away.

Dirty Keto occurs for me more often than not in the midst of a get-away or a café or even merely during times of extraordinary worry at work.

WHY DO WOMEN PRACTICE THE KETO DIET

Not just have ketogenic diets been effectively utilized as a treatment for epilepsy for almost a century, yet it likewise has numerous potential medical advantages, even sound individuals can use.

As Mark Sisson puts it, doing a keto reset re-establishes our "manufacturing plant settings." Which is our capacity to shift back and forth between various types of stored fats for energy, depending upon what's accessible? This adaptability has enabled people to flourish for many years since tracker gatherers didn't generally approach consistent bounty and assortment of sustenance that we have today.

For reasons unknown, this adaptability is significant for wellbeing. The biochemical pathways that ketogenic diets turn on have hostile to maturing impacts and can even destroy numerous advanced sicknesses.

Ketogenic diets give medical advantages by:

- stabilizing glucose and bringing down insulin
- reducing oxidative pressure
- improving the number of mitochondria and making them capacity better
- providing our cells with ketone bodies, which is a cleaner-consuming fuel than glucose

- activating a phone tidy up procedure called autophagy, where the phones stall old and broken parts into reusable supplements
- Activating hostile to maturing and mitigating biochemical pathways.

CHAPTER 2 SIGNIFICANT HEALTH BENEFITS OF A KETOGENIC DIET FOR WOMAN

At the point when done effectively, the ketogenic diet may help:

1. **Improve Metabolic Health from Lowered Blood Sugar**

When we change from burning glucose to burning ketones for energy, the glucose and insulin fluctuate substantially less than when we depend on sugars for energy. The liver can always supply only enough glucose in the blood to prop the mind up.

Settling glucose has numerous medical advantages, including:

- Reducing the risk of metabolic disorder and diabetes
- helping with conditions because of high glucose like polycystic ovarian disorder
- Reducing the weight on the body (because there is no requirement for the pressure hormones like cortisol and adrenaline to step in to keep up glucose). This makes adjusting hormones simpler.
- Reducing and possibly clearing up skin break out (because skin inflammation is an indication of an excessive amount of insulin)

A Note on Blood Sugar

On the off chance that you screen your fasting blood glucose toward the beginning of the day when you are in Ketosis (more on how and for what reason to do that in a piece), know you may experience raised morning glucose because of a flood of cortisol and adrenaline. This is known as "the first light marvel" and should decay to sound levels during the day and improve after some time.

2. Lessen Appetite and Cravings

Its actual ketone bodies can smother craving by following up on the nerve centre in mind. Also, settled glucose can help decrease appetite and nourishment yearnings. Finally, high-fat dinners can animate a hormone that expansion satiety in the gut.

Subsequently, numerous individuals on ketogenic diets find that they are significantly less eager and never again longing for the high-starch sustenance they used to adore. They can even skip suppers or quick for a considerable length of time and won't generally be annoyed by the yearning.

3. Improve Brain Function and Protect Neurons

From numerous points of view, the ketogenic diet is excellent for the cerebrum. Clients report that it improves psychological capacity, hinders the movement of neurodegenerative illnesses, and may even shield from such sicknesses.

Here is a portion of the manners in which Ketosis benefits the cerebrum:

Ketosis Provides a Steady Supply of Clean-Burning supplement or fuel to the Brain

Since the mind is the most energy-demanding organ in the body, it is amazingly touchy to the fluctuation of easy fills. Individuals who consistently experience glucose rollercoasters frequently experience cerebrum-based indications of low glucose, for example, uneasiness and exhaustion when glucose plunges low.

Being in Ketosis can help keep this from occurring. For some, ladies, balancing out glucose has a disposition settling impact.

As indicated by Psychology Today, a few examinations propose that ketogenic diets can help balance out psychological maladjustments, some of the time much more capably than meds. Ketogenic diets lessen the manifestations of uneasiness and discouragement in rodents and mice, while numerous little clinical investigations exhibit that ketogenic diet can help balance out schizophrenia.

Ketosis Supports Mitochondria Health and Reduces Inflammation

Before the revelation of neuroplasticity, researchers accepted that a harmed cerebrum couldn't recover. In any case, by improving mitochondria wellbeing, diminishing inflammation, and animating cell clean up, ketogenic diets can enable a harmed cerebrum to fix itself. In this way, the ketogenic diet is very nearly a supernatural occurrence for some cerebrum sicknesses that were thought of as hopeless.

Studies are developing that ketogenic diets (related to different medicines) can either switch dynamic mind issue or help fix the harm. These incorporate horrible cerebrum wounds and neurodegenerative infections like Alzheimer's and Parkinson's. The Wahl's Protocol additionally uses this advantage of the ketogenic diet to help fix neurological harm from numerous sclerosis.

4. Hinders Aging

Need to hinder the clock? The keto diet may be the one to attempt.

Ketosis Turns on the Anti-Aging Genes

Ketosis, correspondingly to fasting or caloric limitation, turns on a gathering of qualities called Sirtuins. At the point when researchers enact Sirtuins in creatures, they found that these creatures live more. What's more, Sirtuins can help keep you lean and fiery during the day and resting soundly around evening time. More research is hard to know whether this impact is the equivalent in people. However, proof appears to be reliable that investing some energy in Ketosis is gainful.

Ketosis Reduces Oxidative stress

Oxidation is the thing that makes steel rust and apples to turn a dark color when they are presented to air. Inside our bodies, oxidation enables our invulnerable cells to kill off germs and makes us tired by the day's end. Notwithstanding, overabundance oxidation can cause ageing and DNA harm.

By decreasing glucose, Ketosis fundamentally lessens the oxidative worry in the body. Glucose is an oxidizing sugar because uncovered oxygen of glucose can assault different atoms and harm them. These damaged proteins are called propelled final glycation results (AGEs).

Individuals with high glucose will have a lot of AGEs, and along these lines age quicker.

What's more, thinks about show ketosis turns on cancer prevention agent qualities and expands levels of cell cancer prevention agents like glutathione.

Ketosis Stimulates Autophagy (Cellular Clean-up)

Ketosis and fasting likewise initiate an enemy of aging cell clean-up procedure called autophagy (auto = self, phagy = eat). Autophagy is the point at which a cell eats its deficient parts to reuse nutrients and keep the various parts working like new. Also, autophagy can ensure against neurodegenerative illnesses, viral and microorganisms' contaminations, and cancers.

5. Ensure Against Cancer

Everybody has rising cancer cells. However, the cells can form into all-out cancers if the body neglects to murder off them off. DNA harm, inflammation, small cell clean up, high glucose, and powerlessness of the resistant framework to execute rising cancer cells together lead to cancers. Advocates guarantee that ketogenic diets may help forestall cancers by tending to these angles.

Ketogenic diets decrease oxidative pressure and inflammation, animate cell clean-up, diminish glucose and invigorate the cancer-slaughtering resistant reactions. Moreover, ketogenic diets benefit from the way that cancer cells can't benefit from ketones.

Solid cells have the decision to depend on glucose or different powers and whether to utilize the mitochondria. Interestingly, as indicated by the 1931 Nobel Laureate Otto Warburg, cancer cells come up short on the capacity to use ketones for energy. They can create heat by burning glucose and glutamine for energy.

Since the condition of ketosis powers cells to depend on ketones and to utilize the mitochondria for energy, Ketosis bolsters solid cells while starving cancer cells. This mainly is by all accounts valid against the absolute most fatal and hopeless cancers.

Regular Ketogenic Diet Mistakes for ladies

A ketogenic diet has numerous medical advantages. In any case, it is conceivable to commit errors that can obstruct them from accomplishing their objectives.

These include:

1. An excess of Dairy

It is anything but a smart thought to incorporate a ton of dairy in a ketogenic diet because the protein in dairy can deactivate Sirtuin, the counter aging pathway, and make an insulin spike. While spread and ghee (from quality fed sources) for the most part don't cause this impact, high-fat cheeses and substantial creams do. What's more, dairy items can be inflammatory for some individuals.

On the off chance that you endure dairy, at that point appreciate some in your diet, however, don't depend on a liberal measure of cheeses or substantial cream as a wellspring of fat. I, for one, accept that crude, fed, and natural dairy is ideal, yet constrain it in my diet.

2. An excessive amount of Protein

Being in a ketogenic diet is muscle-saving, so you need substantially less protein than you would if you depend on starches or proteins for energy.

Amino acids can be changed over into sugar and consumed as energy. Likewise, high admission of protein can be mood killer the counter aging, and against cancer forms in our cells, so it is ideal for eating merely enough protein on a ketogenic diet.

3. Starving the Good Gut Bacteria

Eating next to no or no starches can kill your great gut microbes. This can't be useful for wellbeing.

Studies have demonstrated that sustenance synthesis influences the gut microscopic organisms significantly more than any probiotic supplements. It is in this manner imperative to sustain your stomach microscopic organisms while you are on a ketogenic diet.

Safe starches can be incorporated as a significant aspect of a ketogenic diet or as an enhancement since it effects affects glucose, so it doesn't upset the condition of Ketosis. Safe starches feed great microscopic organisms in the gut as well as get matured into substances that are helpful for wellbeing. Vegetables likewise contain a ton of fibre that can bolster the gut microorganisms and give a significant wellspring of vitamins, minerals, and phytonutrients. As I would see it, it is essential to eat a wide assortment of non-bland vegetables on a keto diet to ensure gut microorganisms!

4. Eating Too Much

Many medical advantages of the ketogenic diet referenced above are because of enacting our survival qualities. To receive full wellbeing rewards from the ketogenic diet, it is significant that you don't tell your body that there is a rich of sustenance.

It is additionally essential to be in a caloric shortfall on the off chance that one goes on a ketogenic diet to treat neurological ailments or cancers.

If your objective is weight reduction, it is as yet essential to be in a caloric shortfall as just cutting starches alone won't be sufficient for fat misfortune.

5. Not Getting Enough Salt and Minerals

Salt gets an awful rep as unfortunate. However, it gives a significant mineral. Being in Ketosis makes the body discharge increasingly salt, so it is critical to guarantee that to eat additional salt and mineral enhancements as essential.

6. Not Eating Enough Non-Starchy Vegetables

As referenced above, not getting enough fibre from vegetables can starve gut microscopic organisms. The keto diet isn't a meat, egg, and cheddar diet, and however many treat it along these lines. The more significant part of us aren't getting enough vegetables in any case, and this can be a simple snare to get into on a keto diet.

The Ketogenic Diet Is Not Stressful

Keep in mind. However, this isn't about hardship. Or maybe, it is tied in with finding the sweet spot where you feel better and without exorbitant appetite or longing for. Everyone is unique, so it will be essential to test to locate your sweet spot.

The vast majority, including Mark Sisson himself, improve when they generally incorporate some regular wellsprings of sugars (e.g., loads of vegetables) and once in a while add bland starches to their diet.

The uplifting news is, it isn't essential to remain on a ketogenic diet consistently to receive this reward. Our progenitors experienced quick, and blowout cycles, and the body is intended for adaptability. We might have the option to decrease cancer risk, drag out life, improve cerebrum capacity, and advantage from Ketosis generally by being in Ketosis or fasting a couple of days seven days.

Is Keto Good for Women?

When all is said in done, men will, in general, improve on a long-haul ketogenic diet than ladies do. From my exploration and experimentation, ladies can pursue a keto diet, yet with specific adaptions. Most ladies will do well with a recurrent ketogenic diet when they remain on the ketogenic diet more often than not and eat dull starches infrequently to spike calories and carbs.

Ketogenic Diet Cautions for ladies/women

Ketogenic diets are not for everybody. There are a few people who ought to be cautious with the ketogenic diet, or if nothing else ought to do it without restorative supervision. While I understand exceptionally few standard specialists will be knowledgeable in the ketogenic diet, there are online administrations that can combine you with an essential consideration specialist who understands keto in detail.

Type 1 Diabetics

People with type 1 diabetes are subject to insulin infusions to deal with their glucose and are at risk for ketoacidosis, which as a hazardous condition where there are perilously elevated amounts of ketones — a lot higher than a dependable individual in Ketosis can accomplish — in their blood.

Individuals with ApoE3/E4 or ApoE4/E4 genes

ApoE means Apolipoprotein E, which is a protein that transports fats and cholesterol in the body. There are three variations of this quality: E2, E3, and E4. Everybody has two duplicates so that you can have any blend of these variations.

Individuals with two duplicates of the E4 variation (ApoE4/E4) frequently don't react well to immersed fats. These individuals will have exceptionally elevated cholesterol, and it will, in general, keep running in their families. These are a little subset of the populace that must be cautious with the ketogenic diet.

If you have these qualities (here's single direction to test for them), make sure to screen your blood lipids if you somehow managed to go on a ketogenic diet. What's more, center around monounsaturated fats, for example, those found in avocados or olives as opposed to saturated fats or MCT oil.

For any other individual, it is a smart thought to screen your blood tests when you begin with a ketogenic diet.

Pregnant and Breastfeeding Mothers

This is a disputable one the same number of specialists accept that the infant needs starches to create, and numerous mothers need sugars to deliver milk. Notwithstanding, dietician Lily Nichols takes that a sound ketogenic diet is ok for pregnant ladies and that it is simpler to get into Ketosis during pregnancy.

Maybe the best approach is to tune in to your body because each pregnancy is unique. If you jump on a ketogenic diet during pregnancy or breastfeeding, make sure to counsel your human services specialist to guarantee that you do it securely.

Ladies Who Struggle with Irregular Period Cycles / Fertility

Women in Ketosis and fasting can turn on the survival qualities in the body and makes the body endeavour to preserve energy. For certain ladies, this can cause unpredictable cycles and fruitlessness.

A ketogenic diet may help with fruitlessness due to polycystic ovarian disorder since it is mostly brought about by insulin opposition. In any case, the ketogenic diet can exacerbate irregular cycles and barrenness for ladies who battle with it from different causes, including pressure and over-work out.

Quality and High-Intensity Athletes

Lifting substantial things and high-force activities uses starches fundamentally. Numerous quality students and competitors will find that their exhibition drops radically when they are on a ketogenic diet.

If you have been keto-adjusted for quite a long time, your body can, in the long run, adjust to create the sugars you have to fuel these exercises. In any case, if you are generally new to Ketosis and need to perform physically, at that point maybe going full Ketosis may not be such a smart thought.

Step by Step Guidelines to Get Started with A Ketogenic Diet for Women

Another simple method to begin arranging a ketogenic diet, most notably for ladies is to utilize Real Plans. Not exclusively can this feast arranging application channel plans to maintain a strategic distance from most any nourishment sensitivity, it likewise can create a keto-accommodating dinner plan and shopping list.

Getting into Ketosis

Except if you've been eating a paleo or base diet and are relatively keto-adjusted (burning ketones for fuel), it is a smart thought "reset" the body to recapture the metabolic adaptability to go into Ketosis or even remain in Ketosis in spite of eating a few starches. Discontinuous fasting is one practical approach to do this. During a water quick, Ketosis can happen in days rather than weeks or months and regularly continues for some time after the fast.

- Being in Ketosis has numerous medical advantages yet, besides, some potential reactions. To boost the medical benefits, you should:
- Assemble your diet from entire sustenance however much as could be expected (mainly green

vegetables and sound fats like avocado and olives)
- Ensure that you keep up a nutrient-thick diet by including organ meats, vegetables, and some low-sugar natural products in your diet
- Limit protein admission, as ProProteinan even now get changed over into glucose and high protein admissions can contradict the constructive outcomes of a ketogenic diet
- Eat only enough to satiation

Using Tests to Improve Keto Diet Outcomes for ladies

It is conceivable to pursue a low-sugar diet or keto diet and not be in Ketosis. When I've by and by tried different things with Ketosis, I utilized different techniques for testing to ensure my ketone levels and blood glucose levels were inside sound reaches:

Blood Ketone and Glucose Testing

The blood glucose testing and Keto mojo meter is an instrument which tests both blood ketone levels and blood glucose levels. More on this soon in an up and coming post about fasting, yet I testing fasting morning glucose and post-feast glucose at 60 minutes. I likewise tried fasted morning ketones and night ketones.

Breathe Acetone Testing

Another approach to test the body's reaction to nutritional Ketosis is through breath $CH_3)_2CO$ levels. This indicates the body is using the number of ketones. Utilized a Level meter (to test breath $CH_3)_2CO$ levels. This gadget is progressively expensive, however, doesn't require strips so it very well may be utilized all the more regularly. I used it to test my reaction to specific nourishments or practices and to check whether they hauled me out of Ketosis.

Primary concern: What I Do

The keto diet isn't the Atkins diet, or an all-meat diet, or anything close. A solid rendition ought to incorporate a wealth of non-bland vegetables and healthy fats from a different origin.

The more you learn, the more you are persuaded that variety is probably the most significant factor in wellbeing. The ketogenic diet can be a helpful device; however, as I would see, it ought to be cycled and ought to incorporate periodic days with additional starches from great sources.

Frequently explore different avenues regarding keto in the winter when nourishment would have generally been all the rarer and starches harder to discover. During these occasions, most of my plate is still, for the most part, green vegetables, and endeavour to devour a wide assortment of vegetables.

How the Keto Diet works For Different Women

How keto ladies are influenced by a low-carb diet – what befalls hormones on keto, and how to change the ketogenic diet to work best for ladies.

Your diet is one of the most significant parts of your general wellbeing, so before picking a particular diet to pursue, it's critical to know it all you can about it. You may have heard unencouraging things about a ketogenic diet, particularly with regards to ladies following the diet.

Some wellbeing specialists are stating that a keto diet adversely influences a lady's hormones. While your diet and nutrition unquestionably affect your hormones, it's a legend that the keto diet has negative impacts.

Sadly, numerous ladies depend on the verbal exchange or what they read on the web to enable them to settle on choices about their wellbeing, as opposed to searching out better data about keto and how it influences ladies' hormones. Deception can shield ladies from difficult keto, which is tragic because numerous ladies would profit substantially from a ketogenic diet, particularly the individuals who experience the ill effects of conditions like PCOS, endometriosis, or uterine fibroids.

Peruse on to become familiar with how a ketogenic diet can affect your hormones and how you feel every day, and what you can do to make modifications. In this post, we'll talk about the ketogenic diet's effect on hormones, how you feel, and what acclimations to make.

Women Who Can Benefit from a Ketogenic Diet?

Attempting a ketogenic diet could be useful for ladies who are:

- In menopause or going to experience menopause
- Having issues with sex hormones
- Struggling with amenorrhea or unpredictable periods
- Planning on getting pregnant and need to have a reliable pregnancy
- Not accomplishing weight reduction objectives with a low-fat diet

- Frequently gorging on high carb sustenance
- Not getting results with different diets, like paleo

Keto is an incredible alternative for such vast numbers of people, particularly ladies. It's critical to talk about your condition and wellbeing with your PCP so you can get an accurate analysis and get help following any adjustments in your body.

Your Thyroid on a Keto Diet

When your body is in Ketosis, is it awful for your thyroid? No, it isn't – for a couple of reasons. How about we investigate. Low carb diets (the keto diet is low carb) and prohibitive calorie diets bring down the thyroid market hormone known as T3. T3 cells make your different cells go through more energy, and, along these lines, researchers accept that a decrease of the T3 hormone could increase conceivable increment life expectancy – it the two monitors energy and lessens free extreme creation

Both T3 and T4 hormones manage your digestion, body temperature, and pulse. A great part of the T3 in your body tries to ProProteinwhile the remainder of free T3 circles through your blood. In any case, because your T3 levels are lower doesn't imply that your thyroid won't work appropriately. Hypothyroidism is frequently brought about by large amounts of stimulating thyroid hormone (TSH), and lesser degrees of T4 in your blood. Accordingly, the pituitary gland endeavours to attempt to get your thyroid gland to deliver more T4 (which causes large amounts of TSH). In any case, the thyroid doesn't react to the pituitary gland (which produces low degrees of T4). At the point when your T3 is diminished, however, the thyroid is alluded to as "euthyroid," which means a healthy thyroid.

Your Body in Ketosis: the HPA Axis and Stress Hormones

The HPA (nerve centre, pituitary, adrenal) hub is the enormous three with regards to hormonal generation. The nerve center secretes hormones, which speak with the pituitary and adrenal glands and guides them to carry out their responsibilities, creating the hormones they should. Being in Ketosis doesn't wreck this. It does the polar opposite. A good ketogenic diet can increment hypothalamic incitement, which benefits the HPA hub. There isn't any proof that a keto diet adversely influences the HPA pathway. Ketone flagging uses an alternate path that may be considerably progressively effective. Hypothalamic neuropeptides are exceptionally raised in a ketogenic diet. Hypothalamic neuropeptides are incredible at hypothalamic incitement. Ketones can cross the blood-mind boundary, and sign these neuropeptides.

Keto and Cortisol

Cortisol is known as the pressure hormone. At the instance, when your body is under pressure, cortisol will take advantage of your protein stores and creates glucose. Your body would usually utilize this glucose to either keep running from the stress or battle it. As a rule, this would be something to be thankful for. In any case, if your cortisol levels are continually high, and you're always worried, your mind and body get drained. The additional glucose delivered by your protein stores will lift your glucose, and that is nothing worth mentioning for your body. Keep in mind how the ketogenic diet possibly improves the HPA hub? It implies cortisol, which is created inside the adrenal gland, is excellent. When you're in Ketosis, cortisol levels remain low.

Be that as it may, in case you're on a keto diet, and you feel awful, here are a couple of things to remember:

- You're preparing excessively hard – high force interim preparing (HIIT) and a ketogenic diet may not generally blend. In case you're doing high force exercises at least three days every week, it can wreckage up your hormones. If so with you, think about what your objectives are. If you need to pick up bulk or improve your athletic presentation, high power preparing is the thing that you have to do. On the off chance that you'd like to diminish inflammation in your body, get more fit, live more, and counteract infection, at that point a ketogenic diet is a manner in which you need to go. It tends to harm to attempt to keep up both of these, so it's critical to think about which is directly for you genuinely. In the start of beginning a keto diet, it can take some time for the body to alter. During this period, resist the urge to stress about the activity, and gradually increase as you feel increasingly good doing as such.
- You're confining calories to an extreme – if your body isn't getting enough calories, it can chaos up your hormones. Limiting your calories for

significant periods isn't stable. The issue with a keto diet is that frequently, individuals mostly don't feel as eager as they used to, and they aren't getting desires, so they wind up eating fewer calories by and large. Honestly, it very well may be challenging to ensure you're eating enough on a keto diet, so it's imperative to follow what number of calories you're devouring. You may be amazed to see that you're underrating. Figure what number of calories you ought to expend each day, and as much as you might be enticed, don't eat as much as that. Eating short of what you ought to can place your body into "starvation mode," and it will look at last upset your hormones.

- You had hormone issues in any case – on the off chance that you've generally had sporadic periods, unexplained ceaseless cerebral pains or spinal pains, you may have had a hormonal awkwardness in the first place. This should be analysed and treated by wellbeing proficient

What a Ketogenic Diet Can Do to Your Periods/menstrual cycle

On the off chance that you've had a sporadic stream for a large portion of your life, a keto diet may standardize this. If you've been on anti-conception medication and lost your period, or if you have regular amenorrhea (genuine competitors and breastfeeding mothers could recover this), your period could return, substantial to begin.

From the start you may have a more substantial stream, going on for longer than ordinary. When your body acclimates to the adjustments in oestrogen and fat stockpiling, you can anticipate that your period should come back to regular, or even wind up being better. While many PMS indications (spinal pain, skin inflammation, spasms, and so forth) regularly improve, Ketosis doesn't fix swelling. This is the outcome of the flood of oestrogen that occurs during that piece of your cycle.

It's likewise evident that hormones influence your insulin affectability. If your blood glucose floods or drops, it is typical. After your period, it ought to return to ordinary levels.

In case you're ravenous during your period, you have to eat! When you're done ovulating, your body prepares to siphon out oestrogen and progesterone. These hormones can cause hunger. Attempt keto well-disposed chocolate or cake plans, or enjoy bacon or steak.

This is what to do to Keep Your Hormones Balanced on a Keto Diet

Attempt these 11 tips:

1. Eat more probiotic-rich sustenance. This will help hold your gut microscopic organisms under tight restraints.
2. Eat more ProProteinn the three days before your period.
3. Don't stress over your weight during your period. The additional weight is held water.
4. Eat more calcium-rich nourishments. Calcium admission can help with any PMS side effects

you're encountering. Think poppy, sesame, celery, and chia seeds, canned sardines or salmon with bones notwithstanding, almonds, and green veggies like spinach, kale, broccoli, bok choy, and okra.
5. Eat more starches during the tenth, fifteenth days of your cycle, as they are your generally fruitful.
6. Continue to take your cranberry supplements on the off chance that you will, in general, get UTIs. Indeed, they have carbs, yet make them realize that as your body recuperates on a keto diet, you may quit getting UTIs by and large.
7. Keep it non-poisonous. Some excellence items or cleaning items have poisonous synthetic concoctions. These expansion xenoestrogens, which can genuinely awkwardness your hormones. Swap out these items for more beneficial ones.
8. Test your hormone levels. The ones you need to check are your SBHG, estrogen, progesterone, and cortisol blood markers.
9. Manage your pressure. As intense as it seems to be, stress upsets your hormones and should be tended to. Attempt to get seven to nine hours of rest during the evening, start moderate exercise, attempt yoga, reflection, nature strolls, and investing energy with individuals who fulfill you.
10. Don't overlook fiber. If you feel clogged up, get fiber from nuts, seeds, and veggies. Over that drink a lot of water to hydrate your digestive organs.
11. Test your pH levels. Keeping up alkalinity is vital – it improves your bone thickness, brings down inflammation, assists with vitamin assimi-

lation, and encourages you to keep up a substantial weight. On the off chance that your pH is excessively acidic, attempt these keto amicable arrangements – lemon juice or apple juice vinegar (blended in water), mushrooms, spinach, tomatoes, avocado, cabbage, cucumber, kale, jicama, broccoli, oregano, garlic, ginger, celery or green beans

Keep your Diet balanced on Keto

An antacid diet can make them astonish consequences for your body – including against aging, adjusting hormones, bringing down inflammation, and detoxifying. Numerous ketogenic diets will in general pass up this. Before you go keto, it's ideal for reestablishing an antacid pH first, so you don't feel awkward or excessively eager.

A soluble diet underpins your general wellbeing by diminishing side effects related to PMS, menopause, and barrenness by expanding nutrient retention. Eating FOODS that are high in specific minerals; however, not exceptionally acidic can likewise help. The body is ordinarily soluble, yet present-day handled nourishment diets will, in general, make us progressively acidic, which causes an entire host of issues, similar to bone misfortune, muscle misfortune, and a brought down resistant framework. You can test your pH with a pee testing unit. The objective is to in a perfect world have a pee pH level between 7.0–7.5.

When you consolidate a soluble diet with a low-carb diet, numerous ladies experience a decrease in their indications on account of the high nutrient admission, and a brought down measure of poisonous substances. Your diet, be that as it may, isn't the best way to influence your pH level and hormones. Stress, rest and daylight are different factors. - Fasting is likewise an extraordinary method to keep up against aging also and can be substantial. Fasting is especially incredible for post-menopausal ladies, therefore. It enables the body to take a break from stomach related capacities, and spotlight on fixing the remainder of the body. The body's assets go towards re-establishing your cells as opposed to processing. Ladies ought to have a light supper, and then quick for around 13-15 hours among supper and breakfast. You may see enhancements in glucose control and weight. Another alternative is to skip supper a couple of days, seven days. Tea or soup can help check hunger. For most ladies, this is certainly not a major ordeal, except if the lady is dynamic. Have a go at cycling your fasting, so you quick on a few non-successive days seven days. Nowadays, practice just delicately or do yoga, so you don't feel worn out or extra eager.

Think about this as an approach to feel much improved and mend your body instead of a handy solution for weight reduction. Attempt it for a couple of months to test the impacts, and give experimentation to figure a shot what's best for your body. To start with, give centering a shot soluble, and then gradually include fasting and keto.

Precautions to Take before Starting Keto for ladies

Besides the reactions that your body begins encountering while it alters (blockage, desires), you may likewise have awful breath, feminine cycle issues, adrenal or thyroid issues, or low energy levels. While you may feel terrible from the outset, recall that your body needs time to change. These things should clear up in only half a month. Make sure to rest soundly, decrease your pressure, drink a lot of water, and remain tolerably dynamic.

CHAPTER 3 INTERMITTENT FASTING AND KETO DIET

What Is Intermittent Fasting? Clarified in Human Terms

A marvel called intermittent fasting is as of now one of the world's most well-known health and wellness patterns. Intermittent fasting as it is presently comprehended and practice are regularly accepted to have generally in charge of the across the board selection of the diet among working out and figure rivalry circles. In any case, fasting as a dietary standard goes back a lot more remote than that.

It includes substituting cycles of fasting and eating.

Numerous investigations demonstrate this can cause weight reduction, improve metabolic health, secure against illness and maybe help you live more. This Keto diet book for women clarifies what intermittent fasting is, and why you should mind.

Intermittent Fasting Help Loss Fat and Maintaining Muscle Mass

Research has indicated intermittent fasting can be a productive weight reduction device and now and then more compelling than basically cutting calories.

In one investigation, intermittent fasting was demonstrated to be as successful as consistent calorie limitation in battling obesity. In concentrates done by the NIH, there was accounted for weight reduction with over 84% of members — regardless of which fasting plan they picked.

Like ketosis, intermittent fasting builds fat misfortune while keeping up fit bulk. In one investigation, scientists inferred that fasting brought about more noteworthy weight reduction (while safeguarding muscle) than a low-calorie diet, although the complete caloric admission was the equivalent.

The reality is, in case you're attempting to lose fat, doing ketosis and IF can be gigantic assistance. In any case, that is not where the advantages stop.

The Effects of Stress Levels and Cognitive Function on Intermittent Fasting

Fasting has been demonstrated to improve your memory, diminish oxidative pressure, and protect your learning capabilities.

Researchers accept this happens provided that powers your cells to perform better. Since your cells are under mellow pressure while fasting, the best cells adjust to this worry by improving their capacity to adapt, while the weakest cells kick the bucket.

This is like the pressure your body experiences when you hit the rec centre. Exercise is a type of stress your body suffers to improve and get more grounded, as long as you rest enough after your workouts. This additionally applies for intermittent fasting: As long as you keep on shifting back and forth between standard dietary patterns and fasting, it will keep on profiting you.

The majority of this implies both ketosis and IF can help improve your capacity on account of the defensive and stimulating impacts of ketones, just as the mellow cell stress brought about by fasting.

What Is Intermittent Fasting?

Intermittent fasting is an eating design where you cycle between times of eating and fasting.

It doesn't utter a word about which nourishments to eat, yet instead when you ought to eat them.

There are a few distinctive intermittent fasting strategies, all of which split the day or week into eating periods and fasting periods.

A great many people effectively "quick" consistently, while they rest. Intermittent fasting can be as necessary as expanding that quickly somewhat more.

You can do this by skipping breakfast, eating your first supper around early afternoon and your last feast at 8 pm.

At that point, you're fasting for 16 hours consistently and confining your eating to an 8-hour eating window. Here is the most popular type of intermittent fasting, known as the 16/8 strategy.

In spite of what you may think, intermittent fasting is entirely simple to do. Numerous individuals report feeling good and having more vitality during a quick.

Appetite is generally not unreasonably huge of an issue, even though it tends to be an issue to start with, while your body is becoming accustomed to not eating for expanded timeframes.

No nourishment is allowed during the fasting time frame. However, you can drink water, espresso, tea and other non-caloric refreshments.

A few types of intermittent fasting allow modest quantities of low-calorie nourishments during the fasting time frame.

Taking enhancements is, for the most part, allowed while fasting, insofar as there are no calories in them.

Intermittent fasting (or "IF") is an eating design where you cycle between times of eating and fasting. It is a mainstream health and wellness pattern, with research to back it up.

Why Fast?

People have been fasting for a great many years.

Once in a while, it was done out of need when there wasn't any nourishment accessible.

In different occurrences, it was accomplished for religious reasons. Different religions, including Islam, Christianity and Buddhism, command some fasting.

People and different creatures additionally frequently intuitively quick when wiped out.

There is not much about fasting, and our bodies are all around prepared to deal with broadened times of not eating.

A wide range of procedures in the body change when we don't eat for some time, to allow our bodies to flourish during a time of starvation. It has to do with hormones, qualities and significant cell fix forms.

Whenever fasted, we get noteworthy decreases in glucose and insulin levels, just as an exceptional increment in human development hormone. Numerous individuals do intermittent fasting to get more fit, as it is a straightforward and viable approach to limit calories and consume fat.

Others do it for metabolic health benefits, as it can improve different distinctive hazard elements and health markers.

There is likewise some proof that intermittent fasting can enable you to live more. Concentrates in rodents demonstrate that it can expand life expectancy as adequately as calorie confinement.

Some exploration additionally proposes that it can help ensure against maladies, including coronary illness, type 2 diabetes, malignancy, Alzheimer's sickness and others. Other individuals mostly like the accommodation of intermittent fasting.

It is a powerful "life hack" that makes your life less complicated while improving your health simultaneously. The fewer dinners you have to get ready for, the less complicated your life will be.

Not eating 3-4+ times each day (with the arrangement and cleaning included) additionally spares time. A great deal of it.

People are very much adjusted to fasting now and then. Present-day research demonstrates that it has benefits for weight reduction, metabolic health, and ailment aversion and may even enable you to live more.

Intermittent fasting is a dietary way of thinking that uses fasting and devouring periods. There are a few varieties of intermittent fasting with the most prominent fasting convention being a 16 hour quick followed by an 8-hour devouring window.

Intermittent fasting doesn't by configuration recommend explicit calorie distributions, macronutrient proportions, or give a rundown of fortunate or unfortunate nourishments to eat and is commonly not prohibitive of any nourishments.

Meal Timing/Frequency

In contrast to numerous other dietary structures or plans, intermittent fasting depends exclusively on supper timing and dinner recurrence. As commonly suspected of, intermittent fasting generally embraces a 16-hour fasting window, followed by an 8-hour devouring window.

A great many people will expend 1-2 exceptionally enormous dinners during the devouring window, albeit one can consume a few little suppers all through this time. Other fasting draws near, and for example, the elective day quick utilizes a 24 hour quick, followed by an entire 24 hours of devouring.

Confinements/Limitations

Besides the planning confinements and impediments, there are no immovable nourishment limitations of constraints. This is regularly translated as an "anything goes" during the devouring window.

Notwithstanding, by and by, the individuals who accomplish the best outcomes utilizing intermittent fasting ordinarily apply another dietary system, (for example, IIFYM or flexible dieting) to give them some structure to their nourishment consumption during the devouring window.

Does it Include Phases?

Intermitting fasting does exclude any stages in its dietary convention, albeit a few people will experience fasting cycles where they go significant stretches of holding fast to the fasting conventions and afterwards times of ordinary eating.

Who is it best suited for?

Intermittent fasting is most appropriate for individuals who have occupied calendars. And would want to lump their eating into 1-2 dinners every day as opposed to spreading them for the day. Fasting can likewise be astounding for individuals figuring out how to oversee craving signs and retraining their dietary patterns.

Intermittent fasting is likewise a fantastic method to help individuals control calories as regularly shortening the measure of time one eats during the day can lessen in overall calories.

How easy is it to Follow?

Intermittent fasting is anything but difficult to follow in that it doesn't constrain or limit nourishment, allows one to eat without firmly following calories, and won't put weight on your public activity (for example not having the option to go out to supper and request something on the menu). It likewise can make life a lot simpler as there is less time spent cooking, eating, and tidying up.

It very well may be hard for specific individuals who appreciate the way toward cooking and eating; individuals who battle figuring out how to oversee hunger during the early periods of receiving the diet may likewise think that it's hard to follow.

Standard Belief behind Diet

The usual conviction behind intermittent fasting is that it opens parts of our development as individuals and passes on some health and weight reduction benefits when contrasted with our traditional three suppers for each day approach.

A few of the convictions fundamental intermittent fasting are:

1. Maximizing the time your body spends oxidizing fat
2. Minimizing in general insulin burden to the framework

3. Improved vitality levels,
4. Increased life span.

Logical Studies and Interpretation of Data

Many investigations dive into the advantages of intermittent fasting as an instrument to advance fat misfortune.

As referenced earlier, the perfect of fasting to advance health advantages have been around since old human advancement.

Today, vast numbers of the general theories in regards to the public health advantages of fasting as yet seem to be accurate, anyway whether this has more to do with caloric confinement is still easy to refute.

Fat Loss Benefits

One of the significant cases of intermittent fasting is that it is an incredible device for fat misfortune. There have been a few investigations that have analysed the job of supper recurrence in fat misfortune, including things like interchange day fasting and even the intermittent fasting convention.

For quite a while these examinations were dismissed by web-based life and wellness discussions as they were not genuinely investigations of the particular intermittent fasting convention; in any case, as of late one examination was done that followed the customary 16/8 fasting/devouring convention as endorsed by customary intermittent fasting protocols1.

The gathering following the intermittent fasting convention lost about 3.5 pounds fatter than the ordinary dieting gathering; notwithstanding. This additionally happened simultaneously with lower calorie consumption than the typical diet gathering, so it is the more prominent fat misfortune was because of lower-calorie admission.

One of the all the more intriguing notes is that "Testosterone and IGF-1 levels diminished, levels of a few genius provocative cytokines diminished, cortisol levels expanded, insulin and blood glucose levels diminished, triglyceride levels diminished, T3 levels diminished, and RER diminished marginally.

Those are everything you'd hope to find in a calorie deficiency. And know that the facts confirm that the IF gathering was in a calorie shortfall, it was a little one (under 10% below upkeep) – most likely not a massive enough shortage to clarify those impacts.

All in all, this investigation causes it to appear that IF "stunts" your body into believing you're dieting, regardless of whether you're at (or if nothing else near) caloric support, in a way that is commonly steady with improved health and life span".

Muscle Building Benefits

When you take a gander at the fasting writing, it creates the impression that intermittent fasting doesn't seem to pass on any extra advantages to muscle building when calories are held equivalent.

That being stated, times of fasting may improve the nature of muscle tissue by expanding its cell cleaning forms (for example, autophagy and warmth stun protein reaction). Be that as it may, this exploration is right now fundamental and is for the most part theory now.

Health Benefits

Of the considerable number of zones of research on fasting, the impacts of fasting on generally speaking health and life span may be the most fascinating. A few investigations in creature models have demonstrated that times of fasting increment life expectancy and improve a few metabolic parameters as these creatures age.

Maybe the best-known marvels of fasting are increments in autophagy, a cell "cleaning process". There is some excellent creature proof likewise to recommend that fasting may expand life span; in any case, the information in people is present moment, and extended haul information isn't accessible, such a large amount of this is still a hypothesis.

Types of Intermittent Fasting

Intermittent fasting has turned out to be extremely popular in a previous couple of years, and a few distinct sorts/techniques have developed.

Here are the absolute most well-known ones:

- The 16/8 Method: Fasting for 16 hours everyday, for instance by just eating among early afternoon and 8 pm.

- Eat-Stop-Eat: Once or two times per week, don't have anything from supper one day, until supper the following day (a 24-hour quick).
- The 5:2 Diet: This takes off during the two days of the week, eat just around 500–600 calories.

Approaches to Intermittent Fasting

Intermittent fasting has been hugely in fashion lately.

It is professed to cause weight reduction, improve metabolic health and maybe even expand life expectancy.

Of course, given the fame, a few unique sorts/strategies for intermittent fasting have been conceived.

Every one of them can be compelling, yet which one fits best will rely upon the person.

Here are six mainstream approaches to do intermittent fasting.

1. The 16/8 Method: Fasting for 16 hours every day.

The 16/8 Method includes fasting each day for 14-16 hours and confining your everyday "eating window" to 8-10 hours.

Inside the eating window, you can fit in 2, 3 or more suppers.

This technique is otherwise called the Leangains convention. Doing this technique for fasting can be as straightforward as not having anything after supper and skipping breakfast.

For example, if you finish your last supper at 8 pm and, at that point don't eat until 12 early afternoons the following day, at that point you are fasting for 16 hours between dinners.

It is, for the most part, suggested that women quick 14-15 hours since they appear to improve somewhat shorter fasts.

For individuals who get ravenous toward the beginning of the day and like to have breakfast, at that point, this can be difficult to become accustomed to from the start. Notwithstanding, many breakfast captains entirely eat along these lines.

You can drink water, espresso and other non-caloric refreshments during the quick, and this can help lessen appetite levels.

It is imperative to eat, for the most part, healthy nourishments during your eating window. This won't work if you eat loads of shoddy nourishment or extreme measures of calories.

For one to see this as the most "regular" approach to do intermittent fasting. I eat along these lines myself and see it as 100% natural.

Eat a low-carb diet, so that your craving is blunted to some degree. Just don't feel hungry until around 1 pm toward the evening. At that point, eat my last supper around 6-9 pm, so wind up fasting for 16-19 hours.

The 16/8 technique includes everyday fasts of 16 hours for men and 14-15 hours for women. On every day, you limit your eating to an 8-10 hour "eating window" where you can fit in 2-3 or more suppers.

2. The 5:2 Diet: Fast for two days out of every week.

The 5:2 diet includes eating ordinarily five days of the week while limiting calories to 500-600 on two days of the week.

This diet is additionally called Fast food.

On the fasting days, it is suggested that women eat 500 calories, and men 600 calories.

For instance, you may eat typically on all days aside from Mondays and Thursdays, where you eat two little dinners (250 calories for each supper for women, and 300 for men).

As pundits accurately call attention to, no investigations are testing the 5:2 diet itself, yet there are a lot of concentrates on the advantages of intermittent fasting.

The 5:2 diet, or the Fast diet, includes eating 500-600 calories for two days of the week, however eating the other five days ordinarily.

3. Eat-Stop-Eat: Do a 24-hour quick, on more than one occasion per week.

Eat-Stop-Eat includes a 24-hour quick, either on more than one occasion for every week.

By fasting from supper one day, to supper the following, this adds up to a 24-hour quick.

For instance, if you finish supper on Monday at 7 pm, and don't have until supper the following day at 7 pm, at that point you've recently done an entire 24-hour quick.

You can likewise quick from breakfast to breakfast, or lunch to lunch. The final product is the equivalent.

Water, espresso and other non-caloric drinks are allowed during the quick, however no energetic nourishment.

If you are doing this to get in shape, at that point, it is significant that you eat regularly during the eating time frames. As in, eat a similar measure of nourishment as though you hadn't been fasting by any means.

The issue with this strategy is that an entire 24-hour quick can be genuinely hard for some individuals.

Be that as it may, you don't have to bet everything immediately, beginning with 14-16 hours and after that moving upwards from that point is excellent.

Eat-Stop-Eat is an intermittent fasting program with a couple of 24-hour fasts every week.

4. Substitute Day Fasting: Fast every other day.

Substitute Day fasting means fasting each other day.

There are a few distinct variants of this. Some of them allow around 500 calories during fasting days.

A large number of lab studies indicating health advantages of intermittent fasting utilized some form of this.

A full quick every other day appears to be somewhat outrageous, so I don't prescribe this for tenderfoots.

With this technique, you will head to sleep hungry a few times each week, which isn't extraordinarily charming and most likely unsustainable in the long haul.

Exchange day fasting means fasting each other day, either by not eating anything or just eating a couple of hundred calories.

5. The Warrior Diet: Fast during the day, eat a huge meal around evening time.

The Warrior Diet includes eating limited quantities of raw foods grown from the ground during the day, at that point, eating one immense feast around evening time.

Essentially, you "quick" throughout the day and "gala" around evening time inside a 4-hour eating window.

The Warrior Diet was one of the primary mainstream "diets" to incorporate a type of intermittent fasting.

This diet likewise stresses nourishment decisions that are very like a paleo diet - entire, natural nourishments that take after what they resembled in nature.

The Warrior Diet is tied in with eating just modest quantities of vegetables and organic products during the day, at that point, eating one immense dinner during the evening.

6. Unconstrained Meal Skipping: Skip meals when you want.

You don't need to follow organized intermittent fasting intend to receive a portion of the rewards.

Another alternative is to skip suppers every once in a while, when you don't feel hungry or are too occupied to even think about cooking and eat.

It is a fantasy that individuals need to eat at regular intervals, or they will hit "starvation mode" or lose muscle.

The human body is all around prepared to deal with extensive stretches of starvation, not to mention missing a couple of suppers now and again.

So in case you're genuinely not ravenous one day, skip breakfast and have a healthy lunch and supper. Or then again in case you're voyaging someplace and can't discover anything you need to eat, do a short quickly.

Skirting 1 or 2 suppers when you feel so slanted is essentially an unconstrained intermittent quick.

Make a point to eat healthy nourishments at different suppers.

Four hints to keep an intermittent fasting diet on track

As intrigue develops in intermittent fasting, so make the inquiries concerning how to benefit from the weight reduction methodology.

The advantages are clear: the plans can be anything but difficult to follow; some don't require any calorie tallying; they can make individuals healthier and may even defer the side effects of Alzheimer's.

Intermittent fasting likewise doesn't prompt dietary issues or slow down an individual's digestion

Regularly for half a month after the special seasons to shed a couple of pounds. The 16:8 arrangement is less severe than different plans, yet on the off chance that she needs a progressively quick weight reduction, she'll decide on interchange day fasting.

"The initial five quick days are entirely dubious, yet once your body gets changed following that sort of up-down example of eating, it gets straightforward,". So how would you support your odds of intermittent fasting achievement?

First things, first:

Intermittent fasting isn't for everybody, incorporating individuals with sort one diabetes, pregnant women and lactating women. Individuals with overeating confusion will, in general, indulge during their eating window, so this kind of routine won't work for them.

Consider the intermittent fasting plan directly for you:

A portion of the famous regimens include:

The 16:8 diet, or time-limited sustaining, were you quick for 16 hours per day, however, are allowed to eat anything you desire in the other eight hours. Specialists exhort picking an eating window that gives you a chance to complete your suppers genuinely early, for example, 10 a.m. to 6 p.m. or then again prior. In light of the fact that your body is less productive at taking care of sugar as the day passes by.

Substitute day fasting, which means constraining yourself to 500 calories one day, at that point, eating anything you desire the following, and afterwards rehashing that procedure.

The 5:2 arrangement, which means joining two non-back to back quick days into your week, at that point eating typically during different days.

Here are four hints to keep your arrangement on track:

1. **How will I manage hunger during intermittent fasting?**

Eat high-fibre nourishments, for example, nuts, beans, products of the soil, and high protein nourishments, including meat, fish, tofu, or nuts, during your eating window. Biting high-fibre chewy candies can likewise help.

Drink bunches of water. Individuals will, in general, believe they're ravenous when they are exceptionally dehydrated.

Go for dark espresso or tea, or cinnamon or natural liquorice teas. These refreshments may have hunger stifling impacts.

Watch less TV: "I know this sounds weird, yet while you are staring at the TV, you are shelled with many advertisements for nourishment. This can make you feel hungry, when, in fact, you are not ravenous by any stretch of the imagination.

Keep in mind, being "somewhat ravenous" is the best thing that can transpire, health and nourishment editorial manager at NBC News, considering it a "genuine personality body association" that encourages you to perceive completion.

Diet fantasies exposed: Tips to get in shape and keep it off

2. When would it be advisable for me to work out?

Consolidating interchange day fasting and exercise, they allowed the members to pick whether they needed to practice on devouring or fasting day and found there was no solid inclination one way or the other.

What is the OMAD diet? Figure out how the one-supper daily diet functions

That being stated, practice before you eat because individuals get ravenous about 30 minutes after they complete the process of working out and may discover it too painful even to consider sticking to their arrangement if they can't eat anything at all a while later.

In case you're on the 16:8 arrangement, practice previously or during your eating window. In case you're doing exchange, day fasting and are practising on your 500-calorie day, extra nourishment for after your activity session.

3. Is it OK to skip breakfast?

Indeed, the idea that overlooking a morning feast is terrible for your waistline likely started with studies supported by grain organizations. And the more significant part of that exploration took a gander at the impacts of breakfast skipping on discernment in kids, Noted: "I don't know how that all got meant body weight."

Another investigation, by heftiness and sustenance specialist David Allison, found there wasn't relevant information to absolutely bolster a connection between having breakfast and weight reduction and skipping breakfast and weight gain.

4. How would I battle sentiments of low energy or low concentration during fasting?

Have a go at drinking dark espresso: It improves focus and vitality and has no calories in it.

Take a full breath and offer yourself a reprieve: Mindfulness and a touch of contemplation can go far in making you feel better during the fasting time frame.

INTERMITTENT FASTING FOR WOMEN

Intermittent fasting (IF) portrays an example of eating that cycles between times of fasting and typical eating.

Intermittent fasting has turned out to be progressively well known as of late.

Not at all like most diets that disclose to you what to eat, intermittent fasting centres around when to eat by joining ordinary transient fasts into your daily practice.

Along these lines of eating may enable you to expend fewer calories, get more fit and lower your danger of diabetes and coronary illness.

Nonetheless, various investigations have recommended that intermittent fasting may not be as gainful for women all things considered for men. Thus, women may need to follow a changed methodology.

Here is a nitty-gritty tenderfoot's manual for intermittent fasting for women

The most well-known techniques incorporate fasting on substitute days, every day, 16-hour fasts or fasting for 24 hours, two days per week. With the end goal of this article, the term intermittent fasting will be utilized to depict all regimens.

In contrast to most diets, intermittent fasting doesn't include the following calories or macronutrients. Indeed, there are no prerequisites about what nourishments to eat or abstain from, making it to a higher degree a way of life than a diet.

Numerous individuals utilize intermittent fasting to shed pounds as it is a straightforward, helpful and successful approach to eat less and diminish muscle to fat ratio. It might likewise help lessen the danger of coronary illness and diabetes, save bulk and improve mental prosperity. Besides, this dietary example can help spare time in the kitchen as you have fewer suppers to design, get ready and cook.

Intermittent fasting is an eating design that incorporates customary, momentary fasts. It is a famous direction for living that has potential advantages for weight reduction, body synthesis, illness avoidance and prosperity.

Intermittent Fasting Affects Women Differently

There is some proof that intermittent fasting may not be as advantageous for certain women for what it's worth for men.

One investigation demonstrated that glucose control intensified in women following three weeks of intermittent fasting, which was not the situation in men.

There are additionally numerous episodic accounts of women who have encountered changes to their menstrual cycles in the wake of beginning intermittent fasting.

Such moves happen because female bodies are amazingly touchy to calorie limitation.

At the point when calorie admission is low —, for example, from fasting for a long time or too as often as possible — a little piece of the cerebrum called the nerve centre is influenced.

This can disturb the emission of gonadotropin-discharging hormone (GnRH), a hormone that helps discharge two regenerative hormones: luteinizing hormone (LH) and follicle-stimulating hormone (FSH).

At the point when these hormones can't speak with the ovaries, you risk unpredictable periods, fruitlessness, poor bone health and other health impacts. Even though there are no impartial human investigations, tests in rodents have demonstrated that 3–6 months of interchange day fasting caused a decrease in ovary size and unpredictable conceptive cycles in female rodents.

Consequently, women ought to think about an adjusted way to deal with intermittent fasting, for example, shorter fasting periods and less fasting days.

Intermittent fasting may not be as useful for women for what it's worth for men. To decrease any antagonistic impacts, women should adopt a gentle strategy to fasting: shorter fasts and less fasting days.

Health Benefits of Intermittent Fasting for Women

Intermittent fasting benefits your waistline as well as lower your danger of building up various constant sicknesses.

Heart Health

Coronary illness is the primary source of death around the world. Hypertension, high LDL cholesterol and high triglyceride focuses are a portion of the principal hazard factors for the advancement of coronary illness.

One investigation in 16 fat people demonstrated intermittent fasting lowered circulatory strain by 6% in only two months. A similar report likewise found that intermittent fasting lowered LDL cholesterol by 25% and triglycerides by 32%. Be that as it may, the proof for the connection between intermittent fasting and improved LDL cholesterol and triglyceride levels isn't reliable.

An investigation in 40 typical weight individuals found that a month of intermittent fasting during the Islamic occasion of Ramadan didn't bring about a decrease in LDL cholesterol or triglycerides.

More excellent investigations with progressively robust techniques are required before analysts can completely comprehend the impacts of intermittent fasting on heart health.

Diabetes

Intermittent fasting may likewise adequately help oversee and lessen your danger of creating diabetes.

Like consistent calorie confinement, intermittent fasting seems to lessen a portion of the hazard factors for diabetes. It does so mostly by lowering insulin levels and decreasing insulin obstruction.

In a randomized controlled investigation of more than 100 overweight or stout women, a half year of intermittent fasting decreased insulin levels by 29% and insulin opposition by 19%. Glucose levels continued as before. Also, 8–12 weeks of intermittent fasting has been appeared to lower insulin levels by 20–31% and glucose levels by 3–6% in people with pre-diabetes — a condition where glucose levels are raised, however not sufficiently high to analyze diabetes.

Be that as it may, intermittent fasting may not be as gainful for women for what it's worth for men regarding glucose.

A little report found that glucose control intensified for women following 22 days of substitute day fasting, while there was no unfriendly impact on glucose for men Despite this reaction, the decrease in insulin and insulin opposition would in any case likely lessen the danger of diabetes, especially for people with pre-diabetes.

Weight reduction

Intermittent fasting can be an essential and powerful approach to get thinner when done appropriately, as customary transient fasts can enable you to expend fewer calories and shed pounds.

Various examinations propose that intermittent fasting is as viable as conventional calorie-limited diets for temporary weight reduction.

Survey of concentrates in overweight grown-ups discovered intermittent fasting prompted a healthy weight reduction of 15 lbs (6.8 kg) throughout three a year. Another study indicated intermittent fasting diminished body weight by 3–8% in overweight or fat grown-ups over a time of 3–24 weeks. The audit additionally found that members decreased their abdomen perimeter by 3–7% over a similar period. It ought to be noticed that the long haul impacts of intermittent fasting on weight reduction for women stay to be seen.

For the time being, intermittent fasting appears to help in weight reduction. Be that as it may, the sum you lose will probably rely upon the number of calories you expend during non-fasting periods and to what extent you cling to the way of life.

It May Help You Eat Less

Changing to intermittent fasting may typically enable you to eat less.

One examination found that youngsters ate 650 fewer calories for each day when their nourishment admission was confined to a four-hour window. Another investigation in 24 healthy people took a gander at the impacts of a long, 36-hour quick on dietary patterns. In spite of expending additional calories on the post-quick day, members dropped their absolute calorie balance by 1,900 calories, a considerable decrease.

Other Health Benefits

Various human and creature studies propose that intermittent fasting may likewise yield other health benefits.

- Reduced irritation: Some investigations demonstrate that intermittent fasting can decrease key markers of aggravation. Ceaseless irritation can prompt weight gain and different health issues.
- Improved mental prosperity: One survey found that two months of intermittent fasting diminished discouragement and gorging practices while improving self-perception in stout grown-ups.
- Increased life span: Intermittent fasting has been appeared to expand life expectancy in rodents and mice by 33–83%. The impacts on life span in people is yet to be resolved.
- Preserve bulk: Intermittent fasting seems, by all accounts, to be progressively compelling at holding amount contrasted with constant calorie confinement. Higher amount causes you to consume more calories, even very still.
- Specifically, the health advantages of intermittent fasting for women should be contemplated all the more widely in well-planned human examinations before any ends can be drawn.

Intermittent fasting may enable women to get thinner and lessen their danger of coronary illness and diabetes. In any case, further human examinations are expected to affirm these discoveries.

Best Types of Intermittent Fasting for Women

With regards to dieting, there is nobody size-fits-all methodology. This likewise applies to intermittent fasting.

As a rule, women should adopt a more loosened up strategy to fasting than men.

This may incorporate shorter fasting periods, less fasting days or potentially expending few calories on the fasting days.

Here are the absolute best kinds of intermittent fasting for women:

- **Crescendo Method**: Fasting 12–16 hours for a few days every week. Fasting days ought to be non-consecutive and separated equitably over the week (for instance, Monday, Wednesday and Friday).
- Eat-stop-eat (additionally called the 24-hour convention): A 24-hour full quick on more than one occasion per week (limit of two times each week for women). Start with 14–16-hour fasts and continuously develop.
- The 5:2 Diet (likewise called "The Fast Diet"): Restrict calories to 25% of your standard admission (around 500 calories) for two days per week and eat "ordinarily" the other five days. Allow one day between fasting days.
- Modified Alternate-Day Fasting: Fasting each other day yet eating "typically" on non-fasting days. You are allowed to devour 20–25% of your typical calorie consumption (around 500 calories) on a fasting day.
- The 16/8 Method (likewise called the "Leangains strategy"): Fasting for 16 hours every day and eating all calories inside an eight-hour window. Women are encouraged to begin with 14-hour fasts and in the long run, develop to 16 hours.

Whichever you pick, it is as yet critical to eat well during the non-fasting periods. If you eat a lot of unhealthy, calorie-thick nourishments during the non-fasting periods, you may not encounter a similar weight reduction and health benefits.

Toward the day's end, the best approach is one that you can endure and continue in the long haul, and which doesn't bring about any adverse health outcomes.

There are numerous ways for women to do intermittent fasting. Probably the best strategies incorporate the 5:2 diet, changed substitute day fasting and the crescendo strategy.

The most effective method to Get Started

The beginning is straightforward.

Indeed, odds are you've just done numerous intermittent fasts previously. Numerous individuals naturally eat this way, skipping morning or night suppers.

The most straightforward approach to begin is to pick one of the intermittent fasting strategies above and give it a go.

Be that as it may, you don't have to follow an organized arrangement necessarily.

An option is too quick at whatever point it suits you — skipping dinners now and then when you don't feel hungry or don't have the opportunity to cook can work for specific individuals.

By the day's end, it doesn't make a difference which sort of quick you pick. The most significant thing is to take note of a technique that works best for you and your way of life.

The secure method to begin is to pick one of the strategies above and give it a go. Stop quickly on the off chance that you experience any antagonistic impacts.

Safety and Side Effects

Adjusted forms of intermittent fasting give off an impression of being ok for general women.

That being stated, various investigations have revealed some symptoms including hunger, temperament swings, absence of focus, diminished vitality, cerebral pains and awful breath on fasting days.

There are likewise a few stories online of women who report that their menstrual cycle halted while following an intermittent fasting diet.

On the off chance that you have an ailment, you ought to counsel with your primary care physician before challenging intermittent fasting.

The therapeutic conference is especially significant for women who:

- Have a past filled with dietary issues.
- Have diabetes or routinely experience low glucose levels.
- Are underweight, malnourished or have nutritional inadequacies.
- Are pregnant, breastfeeding or attempting to imagine.

- Have ripeness issues or a background marked by amenorrhea (missed periods).

Toward the day's end, intermittent fasting seems to have a decent security profile. However, on the off chance that you experience any issues — such loss of your menstrual cycle — stop right away.

Intermittent fasting may cause hunger, low vitality levels, cerebral pains and awful breath. Women who are pregnant, attempting to imagine or who have a background marked by dietary problems should look for therapeutic exhortation preceding beginning an intermittent fasting routine.

Intermittent fasting is a dietary example that includes ordinary, momentary fasts.

The best sorts for women incorporate every day 14–16-hour fasts, the 5:2 diet or adjusted interchange day fasting.

While intermittent fasting has been demonstrated to be advantageous for heart health, diabetes and weight reduction, some proof shows it might effectively affect propagation and glucose levels in certain women.

That being stated, altered renditions of intermittent fasting seem ok for most women and might be a more appropriate choice than longer or stricter fasts.

If you are a lady hoping to get in shape or improve your health, intermittent fasting is unquestionably an interesting point.

KETO DIET AND INTERMITTENT FASTING IN-DEPTH

Intermittent fasting is what it seems like: not eating for a specific timeframe. Superficially, removing dinners for a set timeframe appears to be flawlessly straightforward. Investigation propels our insight into the best planning for dinners and the supportive changes to our science that happen during fasting.

When you devour carbohydrates, the pancreas starts to discharge insulin-activating carb take-up and capacity.

How Intermittent Fasting Relates to Ketosis?

Intermittent fasting comprises of eating inside a particular encouraging window and not eating the rest of the hours of the day. Each individual, regardless of whether they're mindful of it or not, fasts medium-term from supper to breakfast, for instance.

There are numerous ways to deal with intermittent fasting — a few people quick for 16-20 hours' time spans, on interchange days or following a 24-hour day prompt.

If you need to begin fasting, one prevalent variant is the 16/8 technique, where you eat inside an 8-hour eating window (ex. 11:00 a.m. to 7:00 p.m.), followed by a 16-hour fasting window.

Other fasting calendars incorporate 20/4 or 14/10 techniques. Others practice 24-hour fasts a few times every week.

Intermittent fasting can place you in ketosis quicker because your cells will rapidly devour your glycogen stores and start consuming fat for fuel.

Be that as it may, shouldn't something be said about after you get into ketosis? Is intermittent fasting beneficial reliably?

Short answer: Yes. Here's the reason it tends to be an extraordinary expansion to your health tool stash:

Ketosis and Intermittent Fasting and the Physical Benefits

Keto diet and intermittent fasting are viable devices for:

- Healthy weight reduction
- Fat misfortune — not muscle misfortune
- Balancing cholesterol levels
- Improving insulin affectability
- Keeping glucose levels constant

Ketogenic Diet for Weight Loss, Fat Loss and Improved Cholesterol

The ketogenic diet radically diminishes your carb admission, compelling your body to consume fat as opposed to glucose, making it a viable instrument for weight reduction.

While individual outcomes shift, keto has reliably prompted a decrease in weight and muscle versus fat ratio in a broad scope of circumstances.

In a recent report, subjects who followed a low carbohydrate keto dinner plan altogether diminished body weight, muscle to fat ratio and fat mass, losing a normal of 7.6 pounds and 2.6% muscle to fat ratio while keeping up fit muscle mass.

Mainly, watching the long-haul impacts of a ketogenic diet in hefty patients found that weight and weight of the patients diminished drastically throughout two years. The individuals who radically declined their carbohydrate admission saw a noteworthy lessening in LDL (awful) cholesterol, triglycerides and improved insulin sensitivity.

Comparing a ketogenic diet with eating fewer calories in hefty youngsters and grown-ups. The outcomes demonstrated youngsters following the keto diet lost fundamentally more body weight, fat mass and all-out abdomen circuit. They additionally showed an emotional reduction in insulin levels, the indicator of the Type 2 diabetes.

Intermittent Fasting as a means of Fat Loss and Muscle maintenance

Intermittent fasting can be a productive weight reduction device and now and again more compelling than just cutting calories.

In one examination, intermittent fasting was demonstrated to be as successful as persistent calorie confinement in battling obesity. In concentrates done by the NIH, there was accounted for weight reduction with over 84% of members — regardless of which fasting plan they picked.

Like ketosis, intermittent fasting expands fat misfortune while keeping up slender bulk. In one investigation, scientists presumed that fasting brought about more noteworthy weight reduction (while saving muscle) than a low-calorie diet, even though all-out caloric admission was the equivalent.

The primary concern is, in case you're attempting to lose fat, doing ketosis and IF can be gigantic assistance. Be that as it may, that is not where the advantages stop.

Ketosis versus Intermittent Fasting: Mental Benefits

Past their physiological advantages, both intermittent fasting and ketosis give different mental benefits. Both have been experimentally appeared to:

- Boost memory
- Improve mental clearness and core interest
- Prevent neurological illnesses including Alzheimer's and epilepsy

Keto for Improving Brain Fog and Memory

On a carb-based diet, the fluctuations in your glucose levels can cause variances in vitality levels (referred to as sugar rushes and sugar crashes). In ketosis, your mind utilizes an increasingly reliable wellspring of fuel: ketones from your fat stores, bringing about better profitability and mental execution.

Why? Since your mind is the most vitality devouring organ in your body. When you have a clean and reliable vitality supply from ketones, your cerebrum capacities better.

Also, ketones are better at securing your brain. Studies show ketone bodies may have cancer prevention agent properties that shield your synapses from free radicals, oxidative pressure and harm.

In one examination performed on grown-ups with hindered memory, the ascent of BHB ketones in their blood improved cognizance.

If you experience serious difficulties remaining centred, your synapses might be at fault. Your cerebrum has two first synapses: glutamate and GABA.

Glutamate causes you to structure new recollections, learn confused ideas and gets your synapses to speak with one another. Whenever you content, talk or figure, you can thank glutamate for making a difference.

GABA is the thing that helps control glutamate. Glutamate can make your synapses excessively energized. In the event that this happens over and over again, it can cause synapses to quit working and in the long beyond words. GABA will control and slow down glutamate. At the point when GABA levels are low, glutamate rules free and you experience mental haze.

Implementation of Ketones

Ketones avert harm to synapses by preparing overabundance glutamate into GABA. Since ketones increment GABA and decline glutamate, they help in forestalling cell harm, maintaining a strategic distance from cell passing and improving your psychological core interest.

Ketones help keep your GABA and glutamate levels adjusted.

The Effects of Intermittent Fasting on Stress Levels and Cognitive Function

Fasting has been indicated to improve your memory, lessen oxidative pressure, and save your learning capabilities.

Researchers accept this happens to suppose that powers your cells to perform better. Since your cells are under mellow pressure while fasting, the best cells adjust to this worry by upgrading their very own capacity to adapt, while the weakest cells kick the bucket.

This is like the pressure your body experiences when you hit the exercise centre. Exercise is a type of stress your body suffers to improve and get more grounded, as long as you rest enough after your workouts. This likewise applies for intermittent fasting: As long as you keep on shifting back and forth between standard dietary patterns and fasting, it will keep on profiting you.

The majority of this implies both ketosis and IF can help improve your intellectual capacity on account of the defensive and invigorating impacts of ketones, just as the mellow cell stress brought about by fasting.

Keto and Intermittent Fasting

Carrying on with an LCHF way of life is just eating a higher measure of fat and less sugar to compel the body into a procedure called ketosis, whereby fats are scorched rather than carbohydrates for using as vitality.

A legitimate ketogenic diet requires the dieter to devour high measures of fat at any rate 75%, sufficient means of protein or about 20%, and amazingly low ratios of carbs at about 5% calories.

On the off chance that is eating such low measures of carbs and sugar, you power the body into running on ketones rather than glucose.

Performing intermittent fasting on keto is one of the enormous methods for mending the body and improving health.

Eating a keto diet will make your body to be inclined to utilizing ketone bodies and unsaturated fats as you drive it into ketosis.

In general, it makes fasting easy and a lot simpler for the body contrasted and breaking fasts with high-carb dinners.

Because of expanded satiety on low carb or keto, it is OK with fasting for a long time in succession without getting to be ravenous.

Strategies for Combining Intermittent Fasting with Keto

Generally, intermittent fasting in a ketogenic diet fuses eating a couple of suppers every day, and fasting medium-term and into the early afternoon hours.

You need to eat nourishment exceptionally nutritious and wealthy in nutrients and minerals, for example, natural meat, and vegetables to help fat misfortune.

Eating later in the day or night is significantly more sensible for the vast majority, including me, be that as it may, you should suit it with your way of life.

Pick a timeframe that accommodates your timetable, and you can figure out how to quickly easily.

Here are a few systems that kept running from an 18-hour delayed quick and 6-hour eating window.

Eat between 12 pm and 6 pm, by then, quick from 6 pm to 12 pm the following day.

Or on the other hand, eat between 4 pm and 10 pm, by then, quick from 10 pm to 4 pm the following day.

Radically change this recurrence to suit your needs and increment or lessening the eating window from 8 hours to 60 minutes.

By staying away from that early feast of the day and having only a late lunch and dinner, you are empowering your body to quick for an all-inclusive period.

At the point when drilled over the long haul, it will bolster your fat consuming, muscle building or wellness objectives.

The Perks of Fasting and Doing Keto

The ketogenic diet and intermittent fasting have a considerable lot of similar health benefits. Why? Since the two techniques can have a similar outcome: a metabolic state known as ketosis.

Ketosis has numerous physical and mental advantages, from weight and fat misfortune to improved feelings of anxiety, cerebrum capacity, and life span.

Does intermittent fasting consistently cause ketosis? By no means. If you adopt a progressively mellow strategy to intermittent fasting (for instance, eating inside an 8-hour window), you most likely won't enter ketosis (particularly on the off chance that you eat a high measure of carbs during that window).

Also, not every person who attempts intermittent fasting plans to enter ketosis. On the off chance that somebody who fasts likewise eats high-carb nourishments, there is an excellent shot they'll never enter ketosis.

If then again, ketosis is the objective, and ketones can utilize intermittent fasting as a device to arrive and improve their general health.

Each supper, we eat triggers a metabolic reaction in our body.

Carbohydrates in our nourishment (and to a lesser degree, protein) trigger the arrival of the hormone. The insulin this way advises the body to store any abundance vitality as glycogen or as fat for later use. A portion of the fat is put away in the liver, yet its more significant part ends up fat stores in the body. Insulin starts to discharge fat from fat stores, implying that fat is going into capacity and not utilized as fuel.

When you practice intermittent fasting then again, vitality admission is lower, insulin levels start to fall and fat consuming increments.

By expanding the measure of time the body is in a fasted state, there will be more opportunity for the body to take advantage of putting away vitality. Crosswise over advancement, most species would consistently enter a fasted state. In general, eat more significant parts at a time and may not expend nourishment for a few days. There is nothing amiss with once in a while fasting for longer timeframes, and it has a few health benefits (obviously, counsel your primary care physician before doing this).

Caloric Restriction

Confining the measure of calories, you devour will place the body into a fasted state.

There is a typical conviction that avoiding a supper is terrible for your digestion or generally speaking health. Honestly, we see more information bolster limited eating. The three-dinner daily show has been standard in American diets for a considerable length of time. Stoutness has expanded. Diabetes and pre-diabetes have additionally developed.

Something isn't working.

In studies performed on creatures, those in a fasted state had longer life expectancies contrasted with those that didn't get quick. It appears the advantages of fasting can not exclusively be seen present moment, however through an incredible span also.

An intriguing diet that mirrors fasting is known as the Prolon Diet. The thought is to diminish insulin discharge while as yet giving supplements truly. It's a low-protein, low-carbohydrate, high-fat diet with calorie admission extending from 770 - 1,100 calories for every day. Studies have demonstrated a quick impersonating menu can improve biomarkers for maturing, diabetes and cardiovascular infection.

Points of interest in Intermittent Fasting

Other than advantages for body structure or weight reduction, there are various points of interest of intermittent fasting.

- Easier to oversee than conventional dieting: Preparing a solitary (or a couple, contingent upon your encouraging window) suppers every day is strategically simpler than setting up a few dinners from a period the executive's stance. Also, intermittent fasting spares you the cerebral pain of thorough dinner preparing or discovering nourishments that consent to a particular diet
- The decrease in fat mass: Individuals who rehearsed intermittent fasting demonstrated a lessening in fat mass while keeping up bulk and quality
- Longevity: It is known that populaces who quick all the time can seem to have expanded life span.
- Improved health and digestion: Metabolic health might be improved with fasting by method for circadian science, the gut microbiome, and modifiable way of life practices, for instance, rest.
- Boost mind health: Fasting vigorously is a reliable trigger for neurogenesis and beta-hydroxybutyrate (or BHB, one of the three ketone bodies), which can trigger the arrival of cerebrum development factors.
- Speed up continuance adjustment: Fasting advances pathways associated with fat digestion, which may help perseverance execution—for instance, development of new mitochondria
- Reduced danger of diabetes: Through intermittent fasting, diminished insulin opposition can help those with sort two diabetes lower blood

glucose levels and improve glucose. Intermittent fasting can likewise reduce aggravation.

Useful Application of Intermittent Fasting

Intermittent fasting has been a social column here at H.V.M.N. Workers typically take an interest in intermittent fasting and have referred to higher profitability as one of its advantages, alongside the nonattendance of every day droops related to spikes in insulin from eating carbs. It's not only workers at H.V.M.N. who quick—it's an old-fashioned custom with numerous differences in calendars.

In contrast to numerous different diets, intermittent fasting bargains not with what you eat, but instead when you eat.

This dietary show is tied in with timing as opposed to eating specific assortments of nourishment. When you share in intermittent fasting, you are eating inside a particular window of time. By compelling the body to remain in a fasted state for a more drawn out timeframe, the body will go to fat stores to use for vitality (since it doesn't have carbs).

The body stores much fatter than carbohydrates, and will, in the long run, figure out how to tap into those fat stores for vitality. Just eating in specific windows of time can have a positive long-haul impact on your body synthesis and in general health. Your muscle versus fat can diminish too.

There are various varieties of intermittent fasting, so it's anything but a one size fits all sort of training.

Eating Windows

The most well-known technique for intermittent fasting is picking a specific occasion for nourishment admission (once in a while called "bolstering hours").

You may eat over a four, six, or eight-hour window. This implies you eat during this specific period and the rest of the hours of the day are spent fasting.

A few people quick for 16-hour terms, eating just between the long stretches of 12 pm - 8 pm, and not eating outside of that period. Some do a 24-hour quick consistently. The absolute most committed intermittent fasters will do a 36-hour fast always. Representatives at H.V.M.N. indeed even did a seven-day quick.

Here are two or three different ways to work eating windows and fasting windows into your typical eating plan:

- Four-hour window: the first dinner of the day at 3:00 pm and the last supper of the day is devoured by 7:00 pm
- Six-hour window: the early dinner of the day at 2:00 pm and the last dinner of the day is eaten by 8:00 pm
- Eight-hour window: the first dinner of the day is at 12:00 pm, and the last supper is appreciated by 8:00 pm

A few people may make their fasts a stride further and may decide to eat once every day. This turns into a 24-hour (or close to 24-hour) quick. You should utilize your dozing hours to further your potential benefit, practically like free fasting time (except if you're rest eating). A typical method to do this is to devour your last supper at 8 pm, at that point stand by to eat until 8 pm the following day. Regularly, this is alluded to as one-dinner daily or OMAD fasting.

Notwithstanding the eating window, the complete caloric admission for the day ought to continue as before.

Some may contend that there are points of interest to having a more extended time of fasting, yet your decision of gobbling window is altogether up to you. The best fasting convention is the one that you stick to. Figure out how to function this into your regular timetable generally beneficial, most steady outcomes.

Water Fasts

It's remarkably essential to remain hydrated while you are quick. However, some fasters devour just water during both shorter and longer fasts. Another prominent refreshment decision during a quick is dark espresso. However, this can be viewed as support since it lessens craving.

Substitute day fasting (ADF) is a type of intermittent fasting, however, takes more of an outrageous methodology: no nourishment for 24 hours each other day. Be that as it may, exchange calendars allow for 500 calories to be devoured on fasting days, which have demonstrated to be simpler to stay with.

Regardless of the convention, ADF diets have demonstrated positive outcomes for weight reduction. Strangely, thinks about in creatures showed that ADF may adjust hazard factors for interminable sickness, and can help hold bulk in people (something of a worry with fasting).

Longer water fasts can last somewhere in the range of 36 hours to a few days.

Relating Keto diet and Intermittent Fasting Together

The ketogenic diet and intermittent fasting are categorized to have comparable metabolic pathways thus they ought to have the option to cooperate synergistically

The striking juxtaposition: keto is a type of long-haul dieting with a particular macronutrient focus on, which along with these lines limits what kinds of nourishments you eat. Intermittent fasting happens for a specific time you can eat—with no full scale governs in the eating windows.

Notwithstanding, as investigated prior with low-protein, high-fat, low-carb diets, concentrating on keto during the eating windows may delay the supportive metabolic pathways conjured by fasting. A fascinating application is "Nothingburger," in which he led seven days in length quick between about fourteen days of healthy ketosis.

Both dieting techniques can move in the direction of a similar objective: utilize fat stores for vitality and put the body in a condition of ketosis. Both exhaust the assemblage of glucose. In case you're intermittent fasting, it might have the option to place you into a state of ketosis more rapidly than dieting alone.

. In any case, as our comprehension of the science supporting both develops, we can see clear cooperative energies; this represents the two together can be a decent blend.

Starting a Keto, Intermittent and Hybrid Fasting Diet

Albeit beginning a crossover kind of diet sounds confounded, it tends to be streamlined effectively. Here's a gander at what a single day may resemble in case you're on keto and intermittent fasting. Follow these means for a model keto supper plan that could be utilized while intermittent fasting.

6:00 am: Wake up, drink water or potentially dark espresso.

9:00 am: Drink some espresso in if you're feeling particularly hungry or low on vitality.

12:00 pm: Begin eating window with eight ounces of chicken bosom and a serving of mixed greens with olive oil dressing and feta cheddar. Other lunch increments incorporate hard bubbled eggs, salmon, and avocado.

3:00 pm: Snack on a bunch of almonds and a few blueberries.

6:00 pm: Eat eight ounces of fish joined by vegetables like Brussels grows, string beans or asparagus.

8:00 pm: Blueberries or nuts as a treat, for the last nourishment expended of the day.

In case you're thinking about seven days of intermittent fasting scattered with your keto diet, this is what that week may resemble.

Monday: Feeding hours between early afternoons - 8 pm. In the event that you exercise on Mondays, attempt an early afternoon exercise when you're filled. Make the most of your last supper at 8 pm. Keto suppers may incorporate a smoked salmon and avocado plate, or a steak and sweet potato supper.

Tuesday: Fasting day. No calories devoured until 8 pm.

Wednesday: Try a fasted exercise in the first part of the day. Start eating around early afternoon—you'll presumably be eager. Reward yourself with a significant chicken BLT serving of mixed greens for lunch and cheddar omelette for supper.

Thursday: No exercises, no throughout the day fasting. Since vitality necessities are lesson nowadays, start eating around early afternoon and attempt a turkey, cheddar and avocado wrap for lunch, at that point salmon and asparagus for supper.

Friday: Maybe the fasted exercise turned out poorly way. Today, attempt a workout later in the day, arranging your last 8 pm feast as one high in protein. Attempt simmered chicken combined with rich broccoli.

Saturday and Sunday: Here is another chance to attempt an all-inclusive quick, in case you're groping for it. In any case, in case you're working out, ensure to appropriately fuel until you become entirely fat-adjusted. What's more, use Sundays to feast prep, making the remainder of the week more straightforward!

This is a disentangled variant, however beginning this style of diet doesn't need to be confused. Eat keto-accommodating nourishments in a foreordained window. For this situation, the standard eight-hour eating window was followed, be that as it may, you may observe a shorter eating window if so wanted.

CHAPTER 4- A 14-DAYS KETOGENIC MEAL PLAN FOR WOMEN

Women might have the option to deal with more carbs than keto evangelists guarantee—and may even profit by them in the long haul from a hormonal and vitality yield (for example, wellness) perspective.

Eating low-carb, high-fat incorporates returning to healthy, genuine, natural nourishment. Some have even called it vintage eating. If you like to cook, you'll discover tasty suppers below to make for breakfast, lunch and supper.

Not entirely sure about doing a great deal of cooking? Here are some useful hints to make it simpler:

1. Take a break from breakfast: If you're not ravenous, don't hesitate to skip breakfast and have an espresso (with some milk if you need it).

Numerous individuals find that inside a couple of long periods of eating low-carb, high-fat suppers, yearnings and craving decline fundamentally. This can make it simple to skirt a supper, maybe particularly breakfast.

Skirting a dinner is modest, quick, and might expand the diet's viability for weight reduction and diabetes.

2. Make higher parts: cook two servings and spare the second for lunch the following day. Presently you need to prepare once every day!

3. Freeze remains: Most of the plans stop well, as well, so you can make up a meal, isolate it into littler serving sizes and afterwards solidify some to heat up later for a feast. Maybe you don't need to cook each day?
4. Repeat top choices: Crazy about fried eggs? Love steak? You can eat them regularly.

Assuming, in any case, you discover two or three suppers that you adore, and you find simple, don't hesitate to eat them as regularly as you like. You will get similar outcomes.

5. Necessary no-cook plates: Away from a kitchen or not having any desire to prepare for a feast? Cut shop meats, cheddar, and vegetables with plunge make a simple lunch.

Or then again bubble up twelve eggs and keep them prepared in the cooler to snatch for lunch or bites. A jar of fish or salmon, with some full-fat mayonnaise and vegetable crudités, is a basic lunch.

Smoked shellfish, sardines, herring with crude veggies or a plate of mixed greens are other simple no-cook decisions.

What's more, for women who are ALREADY healthy (for example NOT stout, diabetic or encountering horrendous PMS), long haul low-carb diets as well as not eating ENOUGH fat on a ketogenic diet can be MORE unpleasant—not less—for your body, explicitly your hormones.

Long haul low-carb diets can make you overproduce cortisol and norepinephrine, making an irregularity that expands weight on the nerve centre, pituitary and adrenal organs, bringing about manifestations of HPA-Axis Dysfunction including:

- Difficulty accomplishing a healthy weight
- Less vitality and weakness
- Feeling unrested (regardless of whether you get enough rest)
- Constipation, swelling after suppers and gut issues
- Needing caffeine to feel "typical" or work
- Craving/considering sugar or carbs
- Insatiable hunger or complete absence of desire (unevenness)
- Anxiety, stress or low state of mind
- Poor rest
- Poor exercise results or recuperation
- Amenorrhea or unpleasant PMS
- Not feeling like your "self."

Low carbohydrate diets can likewise affect the hormone Leptin—fundamental for turning ON regenerative hormone work (like your period). Regardless of whether you ARE eating enough fat, leptin is turned on via carbohydrate digestion, and in the long haul might be diminished through an exceptionally low carb admission.

Nobody Size Fits All

There truly is NO one-size-fits-all way to deal with diet.

A few women flourish off deficient carb diets, while others lose their period, or even put on weight after an underlying rest. Everything relies upon TONS of other ways of life elements like:

- Your individual health history
- Sleep and recuperation propensities
- Your feelings of anxiety in different territories
- Body organization
- Hormonal or thyroid lopsided characteristics
- Gut health
- And past

On the off chance that you have a bacterial abundance, for example in your gut, at that point keto conceivably can intensify the condition, as stomach microscopic organisms entirely feed off ketones. If you are doing much work, and dozing under 6 hours of the night, at that point you frequently raised cortisol levels might be MORE worried by keto on the off chance that you keep it up long haul. On the off chance that you were eating sugar or a low-fat diet previously, at that point, your body will presumably LOVE keto—a night and day distinction from prior.

You are NOT frail for going keto for a transient reset, at that point changing back to an altered keto (including somewhat more carb). What's more, you are NOT reliable for "staying with keto" (even though it appears as though your body isn't reacting positively).

Basically: Listen to your body.

Keto Reset: 7-30 Days

Higher Fat with an assortment of healthy fats (going for 50-60% of admission being from fat)

Moderate Sustainable Protein

Lots of Greens and Low-starch veggies for their carbs, adhering to 20-30 grams of "net carbs")

Changed Keto—Longer Term

Eat adjusted at every supper:

Healthy Fats with Each Meal (1-2 servings, and VARIETY—not spread merely, coconut oil and bacon each supper)

Supportable proteins (the size of 1-2 palms of your hand)

Loads of Vegetables

Boring Carbs/Fruit (Incorporate around 1-2 extra servings of bland carbohydrate and additionally natural product once again into your diet every day

The best part? No tallying or ketone is checking important.

When my customers arrive at the Modified Keto organize, 7 to 30 days after the fact, and are re-presenting carbs, they are MORE associated with their body and how it feels—frequently.

They perceive when "cerebrum mist" sets in, or their SIBO side effects (swelling) flares, or when they have a feeling that they have significantly more vitality and quality in their day by day life. They are better ready to self-control the without flaw measure of carbohydrate and timing for their body (for example in the night time before bed, or after an exercise).

It won't come medium-term, yet on the off chance that you adhere to the way of thinking of "equalization" and check out HOW YOUR BODY FEELS, rather than what you "ought to eat" or what your keto screen says, your body won't guide you wrong.

Here's an example 14-day keto feast plan including:

Seven days of a "Severe" Keto (low carb) test

Seven days of an "Altered" Keto test

• Daily supplement plan

Keto Plan Support Supplements

• Soil Based Probiotic: (like Primal Blueprint Probiotics).

Healthy gut microscopic organisms to lift gut and all-around health. Take one toward the beginning of the day and ideally one during the evening. Likewise, don't disregard matured nourishments (like sauerkraut and aged veggies for nourishment based lactic corrosive probiotics).

• Pre-Biotic Fiber: Partially Hydrolyzed Guar Gum (like Sunfiber)

Prebiotics are necessary fibre for assimilation and maximal retention of your probiotics. (Frequently low on a keno-diet). Take one serving/day in water or tea.

• Digestive Enzymes

Supportive for completely separating you nourishment (particularly on the off chance that you experience swelling or stoppage around dinners). Take 1-2 with dinners to expel swelling.

• Bile Salts: Beta TCP

I sit normal to say that you are entirely processing your fats? If your gallbladder or liver is not fit as a fiddle, fats may make you feel wiped out or feelings of queasiness in the wake of eating them. Take 1-2 containers with dinners.

• Fermented Cod Liver Oil: Rosita

Omega 3's, Vitamin A and Vitamin D—fundamental for vitality and retention of all the healthy fats you eat. Take one tablespoon. /day. Unlike most fish oils, old cod liver oil is more averse to go bad.

14 DAYS MEAL PLAN

WEEK 1

DAY 1 MORNING

Smaller than expected Crustless Quiches; Calories: 382, 28F, 22P, 5.3C

Ingredients

• 14 enormous eggs • 3 plum tomatoes, diced • ⅔ cup mozzarella cheddar, destroyed • ⅓ cup pepper jack cheddar, destroyed • ⅓ cup sweet onion, diced • ⅓ cup cut salted jalapenos • ⅔ cup s

Guidelines

1. Preheat the grill to 325°F and oil a 15" x 11" biscuit tin.
2. Consolidate every one of the ingredients in a blending bowl, season with salt and pepper and whisk well.
3. Split the quiche hitter into the biscuit tin similarly and prepare for around 25 minutes.
4. Store in the ice chest and warm when prepared to eat.
5. Sustenance depends on 4 Mini Crustless Quiches. The formula makes about 12.oppressa-tasalami, diced • ⅓ cup substantial cream

DAY 1 LUNCH

Ham and Cheddar Wraps Calories: 600, 44F, 27P, 8C

Ingredients •

1 low carb wrap • 2 table spoon mayonnaise • 2 oz. Cheddar, destroyed • 2 oz. store ham • Pickles or jalapenos to taste • Salt, pepper

Guidelines

1. Onto a low carb wrap, spread the mayonnaise.
2. Include the destroyed cheddar and ham cuts.
3. If you need, including a few pickles or jalapenos for something crisp and delicious.
4. Wrap it up tight and slice it to accommodate your lunch pack or appreciate immediately!

DAY 1 DINNER

Chicken and Mushrooms

Ingredients • 6 oz. chicken bosom • 8 oz. white mushrooms • 2 table spoon margarine • ¼ cup water • ¼ cup overwhelming cream • 1 table spoon crisp lemon juice • Salt, pepper • 1 bunch of spinach

Directions

1. Cook the chicken on a container until it's nearly cooked the whole distance. At that point, let it lay on a plate while you set up the sauce.
2. On that equivalent container, cook the mushrooms in spread until they've contracted and crisped up.
3. Include the water, lemon juice and overwhelming cream and let that cook until the sauce has thickened.
4. Seasoning with salt and pepper and the chicken back in to cook the remainder of the way. Present with a side of spinach.

DAY 2 'MORNING

Scaled-down Crustless Quiches

Ingredients • 14 enormous eggs • 3 plum tomatoes, diced • ⅔ cup mozzarella cheddar, destroyed • ⅓ cup pepper jack cheddar, destroyed • ⅓ cup sweet onion, diced • ⅓ cup cut salted jalapenos • ⅔ cup soppressata salami, diced • ⅓ cup overwhelming cream

Guidelines

1. Preheat the grill to 325°F and oil a 15" x 11" biscuit tin.

2. Consolidate every one of the ingredients in a blending bowl, season with salt and pepper and whisk well.
3. Split the quiche hitter into the biscuit tin similarly and prepare for around 25 minutes.
4. Store in the cooler and warm when anticipated to eat.
5. Nourishment depends on 4 Mini Crustless Quiches

DAY 2 LUNCH

BLT Avocado Wraps

Ingredients • 3 lettuce leaves • 3 table spoon mayonnaise • 6 strips bacon, cooked • ½ Roma tomato, cut • ½ avocado, cut • Salt and pepper

Guidelines

1. Delicately smooth the lettuce leaves and spread a tablespoon of mayo onto each.
2. Lay 2 bacon strips onto each leaf followed by the cut tomato and avocado.
3. Season with salt and pepper.
4. Wrap everyone up firmly and appreciate!

DAY 2 DINNER

Low Carb Chicken Quesadilla

Ingredients • 1low carb wrap • 3oz. Pepper jack cheddar destroyed • 2.5oz. chicken breast, grilled, crushed • ½ avocado, sliced flimsy • 1table spoonchopped jalapeño • ¼ table spoon salt

Guidelines

1. Spot the wrap on a skillet wide enough to allow the wrap to lay as completely level as conceivable on medium warmth.
2. Following 2 minutes, flip the fold around and start spreading out the pepper jack. Try not to get excessively near the corners (leave somewhat less than in inch from the edges of the wrap). 3. Include the chicken bosom, avocado and jalapeño to one portion of the wrap.
3. Overlay the fold around with a spatula and press down to smooth (not all that much!). This will guarantee the liquefied cheddar sticks the quesadilla together.
4. Remove the dish and cut into thirds. Appreciate with salsa and additionally sharp cream!

DAY 3 BREAKFAST

Small scale Crustless Quiches

Ingredients • 14 enormous eggs • 3 plum tomatoes, diced • ⅔ cup mozzarella cheddar, destroyed • ⅓ cup pepper jack cheddar, destroyed • ⅓ cup sweet onion, diced • ⅓ cup cut salted jalapenos • ⅔ cup soppressata salami, diced • ⅓ cup substantial cream

Guidelines

1. Preheat the grill to 325°F and oil a 15" x 11" biscuit tin.

2. Join every one of the ingredients in a blending bowl, season with salt and pepper and whisk well.
3. Split the quiche hitter into the biscuit tin similarly and prepare for around 25 minutes.
4. Store in the refrigerator and warm when made to eat.
5. Sustenance depends on 4 Mini Crustless Quiches

DAY 3 LUNCH

Simple Cobb Salad

Ingredients • 1 large hard-bubbled egg • 4 oz. chicken bosom • 1 cup spinach • 2 strips bacon • ¼ avocado • 1 table spoon olive oil • ½ table spoon white vinegar

Guidelines

1. Carry a pot of water to bubble and cook the egg for 10 minutes. When it's cooked, cool it in virus water and hack it up.
2. On a skillet, cook the chicken bosom and bacon to wanted freshness.
3. Generally, slash or tear spinach leaves and include the bacon, chicken and hacked egg.
4. Toss into equal parts avocado and blend to split it up.
5. Dress with olive oil and vinegar or utilize a low carb Bleu cheddar dressing.

DAY 3 DINNER

Cheddar Chicken and Broccoli Casserole

Ingredients • 20 oz. Chicken bosom, destroyed • 2 cups broccoli florets (we utilized solidified) • 2 table spoon olive oil • ½ cup harsh cream • ½ cup substantial cream • Salt, pepper • 1 table spoon oregano • 1 cup cheddar, destroyed • 1 oz. pork skins, squashed

Guidelines

1. Preheat the broiler to 450°F.
2. In a deep blending bowl, join chicken, broccoli florets, olive oil and sour cream. Blend to merge ultimately.
3. Spot the blend into a lubed 8x11" preparing a dish, squeezing into an even layer.
4. Sprinkle substantial cream over the whole layer. Season with salt, pepper and oregano.
5. Add the cheddar to the top and include the squashed pork skins over the cheddar for a fresh goulash top.
6. Prepare for around 20-25 minutes.
7. Sustenance is per ¼ of the meal.

DAY 4 BREAKFAST

Breakfast (makes 3 servings) Chocolate Peanut Butter Muffins

Ingredients • 1 cup almond flour • ½ cup erythritol • 1 table spoon baking powder • 1 squeeze salt • ⅓ cup nutty spread • ⅓ cup almond milk • 2 huge eggs • ½ cup SF chocolate chips

Directions

1. Consolidate all the dry ingredients (except for chocolate chips) in an enormous blending bowl and mix.
2. Include the nutty spread and almond milk and blend to join.
3. Include 1 egg at once, fusing each completely.
4. Overlap in the SF chocolate chips.
5. Shower a biscuit tin and include the hitter. Prepare for around 15 minutes at 350°F.
6. This formula makes 6 biscuits, 2 biscuits for every serving.
7. Nourishment is per 2 Chocolate Peanut Butter Muffins.

DAY 4 LUNCH

Fish Avocado Salad

Ingredients • 4 oz. canned fish • ½ stalk celery, diced • ½ avocado • 2 table spoon mayonnaise • 1 table spoon mustard • ½ table spoon new lemon juice • Salt, pepper • 1 hard-bubbled egg, stripped, slashed

Directions

1. Join the fish, celery and avocado.
2. Include mayo, mustard, lemon squeeze and flavours.
3. Add the egg to the fish plate of mixed greens.
4. Blend very well until every one of the ingredients is all around joined.
5. Pack it up and spare it for lunch!

DAY 4 DINNER

Cheddar Chicken and Broccoli Casserole

Ingredients • 20 oz. Chicken bosom, destroyed • 2 cups broccoli florets (we utilized solidified) • 2 table spoon olive oil • ½ cup acrid cream • ½ cup overwhelming cream • Salt, pepper • 1 table spoon oregano • 1 cup cheddar, destroyed • 1 oz. pork skins, squashed

Guidelines

1. Preheat the stove to 450°F.
2. In a profound blending bowl, consolidate chicken, broccoli florets, olive oil and harsh cream. Blend to combine altogether.
3. Spot the blend into a lubed 8x11" preparing the dish, squeezing into an even layer.
4. Shower overwhelming cream over the whole layer. Season with salt, pepper and oregano.
5. Add the cheddar to the top and include the squashed pork skins over the cheddar for a firm goulash top.
6. Heat for around 20-25 minutes. 7. Sustenance is per ¼ of the meal.

DAY 5 BREAKFAST

Chocolate Peanut Butter Muffins; Calories: 530, 41F, 15P, 4.5C

Ingredients • 1 cup almond flour • ½ cup erythritol • 1 table spoon baking powder • 1 squeeze salt • ⅓ cup nutty spread • ⅓ cup almond milk • 2 huge eggs • ½ cup SF chocolate chips

Guidelines

1. Consolidate all the dry ingredients (except chocolate chips) in an enormous blending bowl and mix.
2. Include the nutty spread and almond milk and mix to consolidate.
3. Include 1 egg at once, consolidating each completely.
4. Overlap in the SF chocolate chips.
5. Shower a biscuit tin and include the player. Prepare for around 15 minutes at 350°F.
6. This formula makes 6 biscuits, 2 biscuits for every serving.
7. Nourishment is per 2 Chocolate Peanut Butter Muffins.

DAY 5 LUNCH

Cheddar Chicken and Broccoli Casserole; Calories: 548, 42F, 44P, 4C

Ingredients • 20 oz. Chicken bosom, destroyed • 2 cups broccoli florets (we utilized solidified) • 2 table spoon olive oil • ½ cup harsh cream • ½ cup substantial cream • Salt, pepper • 1 table spoon oregano • 1 cup cheddar, destroyed • 1 oz. pork skins, squashed

Guidelines

1. Preheat the broiler to 450°F.
2. In a profound blending bowl, join chicken, broccoli florets, olive oil and harsh cream. Blend to join altogether.
3. Spot the blend into a lubed 8x11" heating dish, squeezing into an even layer.
4. Sprinkle overwhelming cream over the whole layer. Season with salt, pepper and oregano. 5.

Add the cheddar to the top and include the squashed pork skins over the cheddar for a fresh dish top.
5. Heat for around 20-25 minutes.
6. Sustenance is per ¼ of the goulash.

DAY 5 DINNER

Shrimp and Mushroom Zoodles;

Ingredients • 1 table spoon olive oil • 8 oz. white mushrooms, cut • 1 table spoon butter • 6 oz. enormous shrimp, stripped • 1 huge zucchini • ¼ cup marinara sauce • Salt, pepper • 2 table spoon Parmesan cheddar

Guidelines

1. Warmth the olive oil in an massive dish over medium heat. 2. Fry the mushrooms until they've absorbed a large portion of the oil. 3. Include margarine and let the mushrooms cook until they've turned brilliant. 4. Include the shrimp and let them cook for around few minutes on both side. 5. When the shrimp are cooked and pink, hurl the zoodles in for around 2 minutes. 7. At that point, include the marinara sauce and season with salt and pepper. 8. Appreciate with a sprinkle of Parmesan!

DAY 6 BREAKFAST

Chocolate Peanut Butter Muffins

Ingredients • 1 cup almond flour • ½ cup erythritol • 1 table spoon baking powder • 1 squeeze salt • ⅓ cup nutty spread • ⅓ cup almond milk • 2 enormous eggs • ½ cup SF chocolate chips

Guidelines 1. Join all the dry ingredients (aside from chocolate chips) in a huge blending bowl and mix. 2. Include the nutty spread and almond milk and mix to join. 3. Include 1 egg at once, consolidating each completely. 4. Crease in the SF chocolate chips. 5. Shower a biscuit tin and include the player. Heat for around 15 minutes at 350°F. 6. This formula makes 6 biscuits, 2 biscuits for each serving. 7. Sustenance is per 2 Chocolate Peanut Butter Muffins.

DAY 6 LUNCH

Cheddar Chicken and Broccoli Casserole

Ingredients • 20 oz. Chicken bosom, destroyed • 2 cups broccoli florets (we utilized solidified) • 2 table spoon olive oil • ½ cup acrid cream • ½ cup overwhelming cream • Salt, pepper • 1 table spoon oregano • 1 cup cheddar, destroyed • 1 oz. pork skins, squashed

Directions

1. Preheat the stove to 450°F. 2. In a profound blending bowl, consolidate chicken, broccoli florets, olive oil and harsh cream. Blend to join ultimately. 3. Spot the blend into a lubed 8x11" preparing the dish, squeezing into an even layer. 4. Sprinkle substantial cream over the whole layer. Season with salt, pepper and oregano. 5. Add the cheddar to the top and include the squashed pork skins over the cheddar for a firm goulash top. 6. Prepare for around 20-25 minutes. 7. Nourishment is per ¼ of the goulash.

DAY 6 DINNER

Sriracha Lime Flank Steak

Ingredients • 7 oz. asparagus • 8 oz. flank steak • Salt, pepper • Sriracha Lime Sauce: • ½ lime • 1 table spoon sriracha • ½ table spoon vinegar • Salt, pepper • 1 table spoonolive oil

Directions

1. Trim the finishes off the asparagus and let them fry on medium warmth for around 10 minutes, hurling every so often. 2. Carefully seasoned the steak with salt and pepper. Cook for 5 minutes on each side for medium-uncommon. Include 1 moment each side for medium and 2 minutes for well-done. 3. Spread the steak and let rest for 5 minutes. Then, crush new lime in a bowl and blend with sriracha, vinegar, salt and pepper. While whisking these together, slowly pour in olive oil to make an emulsion and thicken the sauce. 4. Cut steak meagre and present with sauce and the asparagus.

DAY 7 BREAKFAST

Smooth Scrambled Eggs

Ingredients • 4 huge eggs • 2 table spoon spread • 4 strips bacon • 2 table spoon acrid cream • ½ table spoon salt • ¼ table spoon dark pepper • 1 stalk green onion

Directions

1. Break eggs and add the spread to a container on medium-high heat. Blend consistently with a silicone spatula. 2. While mixing the eggs, let some bacon strips cook

in another dish (or heat them). 3. Substitute mixing the eggs on the warmth and of the warmth in 30-second interims. When they're nearly done, turn the warmth off. The eggs will keep cooking somewhat more from the leftover heat from the skillet. 4. Include a tablespoon of sour cream and season with salt and pepper. 5. Enhancement with cleaved green onion and appreciate.

DAY 7 LUNCH

Chicken Zoodle Soup

Ingredients • 2 table spoon olive oil • ½ white onion, hacked • 1 medium carrot, cleaved • 1 stalk celery, slashed • 1 table spoon dried oregano • 1-quart chicken juices • 8 oz. boneless, skinless chicken thighs • 1 huge zucchini • ¼ cup harsh cream

Directions

1. Heat olive oil over medium warmth and cook onion and cook until translucent. 2. Include carrots and celery and season with salt, pepper and oregano. Cook until mollified somewhat. 3. Include the chicken juices and heat the blend to the point of boiling. At that point lower the warmth to a stew, include chicken and cook 30 minutes. 4. Expel the chicken thighs and shred them. Cook them for 15 additional minutes. 5. Spiralize the zucchini into flimsy noodles and add them to the soup during the last 2 or 3 minutes of cooking. Appreciate the soup with acrid cream! 6. Nourishment is for 1/3 of the formula.

DAY 7 DINNER

Bunless Butter Burger

Ingredients • 4 oz. ground hamburger • Salt, pepper • 1 table spoon paprika • 1 table spoon butter • 1 table spoon olive oil • 1 enormous leaf of lettuce • 1 cut cheddar • 1 table spoon mayonnaise

Guidelines

1. Season the ground hamburger with salt, pepper and paprika and blend very well with your hands.

2. Make 2 level patties and spot the spread in the focal point of one of the parties. 3. Spot the subsequent patty over the buttered patty and press and seal the sides until the two patties blend. 4. Cook the patty on a skillet with the olive oil on high heat for 4 minutes on each side. 5. When it's set, place the patty on a lettuce leaf and include a cut of cheddar. Spread with some mayo, overlay and appreciate.

WEEK 2

DAY 1

Smooth Coffee Shake

Ingredients • 1 mug blended espresso • ¼ cup substantial cream • 1 table spoon coconut oil • 1 scoop vanilla protein powder (around 30 grams)

Directions

1. Add the prepared espresso to a blender or Nutribullet. 2. To it, include the substantial cream, coconut oil, and the protein powder. We suggest a low carb one like Isopure or NowFoods . 3. Mix on high for around 20 sec-

onds. 4. Be cautious opening the blender as the hot espresso may have made a ton of steam. 5. Appreciate warm!

DAY 1 LUNCH

Chicken Zoodle Soup

Ingredients • 2 table spoon olive oil • ½ white onion, slashed • 1 medium carrot, hacked • 1 stalk celery, cleaved • 1 table spoon dried oregano • 1-quart chicken juices • 8 oz. boneless, skinless chicken thighs • 1 enormous zucchini • ¼ cup sharp cream

Guidelines

1. Warm the olive oil over medium warmth and cook onion and cook until translucent. 2. Include carrots and celery and season with salt, pepper and oregano. Cook until mollified marginally. 3. Include the chicken stock and heat the blend to the point of boiling. At that point lower the warmth to a stew, include chicken and cook 30 minutes. 4. Evacuate the chicken thighs and shred them. Cook them for 15 additional minutes. 5. Spiralize the zucchini into slim noodles and add them to the soup during the last 2 or 3 minutes of cooking. Appreciate the soup with harsh cream! 6. Sustenance is for 1/3 of the formula.

DAY 1 DINNER

Low Carb Chicken Quesadilla

Ingredients • 1low carb wrap • 3oz. Pepper jack cheddar destroyed • 2.5oz. chicken breast,grilled, crushed • ½ avocado, sliced dainty • 1table spoonchopped jalapeño • ¼ table spoon salt

Guidelines

1. Spot the wrap on a skillet wide enough to allow the wrap to lay as completely level as conceivable on medium warmth. 2. Following a 2 minutes, flip the fold around and start spreading out the pepper jack. Try not to get excessively near the corners (leave somewhat less than in inch from the edges of the wrap). 3. Include the chicken bosom, avocado and jalapeño to one portion of the wrap. 4. Overlay the fold around with a spatula and press down to smooth (not all that much!). This will guarantee the liquefied cheddar sticks the quesadilla together. 5. Remove the dish and cut into thirds. Appreciate with salsa as well as harsh cream!

DAY 2 BREAKFAST

Exemplary Steak and Eggs

Ingredients • 1 table spoon olive oil • 4 oz. sirloin • 1 table spoon butter • 3 huge eggs • Salt, pepper • ½ avocado

Guidelines

1. In a container with the olive oil, cook the sirloin (or your preferred cut of steak) until wanted doneness. 2. In the interim, liquefy the margarine in a dish and fry the eggs until the whites are set and yolk is to wanted doneness. Season with salt and pepper. 3. Take the steak off the skillet, cut it into scaled-down strips and season with

salt and pepper. 4. Cut up and salt the avocado and serve everything together.

DAY 2 LUNCH

Chicken Zoodle Soup

Ingredients • 2 table spoon olive oil • ½ white onion, slashed • 1 medium carrot, hacked • 1 stalk celery, cleaved • 1 table spoon dried oregano • 1-quart chicken juices • 8 oz. boneless, skinless chicken thighs • 1 huge zucchini • ¼ cup acrid cream

Guidelines 1. Warm the olive oil in a pot over medium warmth and cook onion and cook until translucent. 2. Include carrots and celery and season with salt, pepper and oregano. Cook until mellowed marginally. 3. Include the chicken juices and heat the blend to the point of boiling. At that point lower the warmth to a stew, include chicken and cook 30 minutes. 4. Expel the chicken thighs and shred them. Cook them for 15 additional minutes. 5. Spiralize the zucchini into slender noodles and add them to the soup during the last 2 or 3 minutes of cooking. Appreciate the soup with sharp cream! 6. Sustenance is for 1/3 of the formula.

DAY 2 DINNER

Mustard Lemon Pork and Green Beans

Ingredients • 2 4-oz. pork flanks • 1 table spoon olive oil • 1 cup green beans • Mustard Sauce • ¼ cup chicken juices • 2 table spoon substantial cream • ½ table spoon apple juice vinegar • ¼ lemon • ½ table spoon mustard

Guidelines

1. Pat pork flanks dry with a paper towel and season with salt and pepper. 2. On an enormous dish with olive oil on high heat, singe the pork on the two sides for 2 minutes. 3. Put them in a safe spot and deglaze the dish with chicken soup, apple juice vinegar and substantial cream. Let this go to a stew. 4. Include the lemon juice, mustard and mix to consolidate. Add pork midsections back to the container and flip once to cover them in the sauce. 5. Give them a chance to cook for 10 minutes with the top of the skillet left marginally open. 6. Dish greens beans in a 350°F stove for 10 minutes and serve together with sauce on top.

DAY 3 BREAKFAST

Pepperoni Pizza Omelette

Ingredients • 3 huge eggs • 1 table spoon heavy cream • ½ oz. pepperoni cuts • ½ cup destroyed mozzarella • Salt, pepper, basil • 2 portions of bacon

Directions

1. Warmth a little container with some oil on a medium fire. At the same time, fry the bacon strips in another dish (or prepare them). 2. Beat eggs with overwhelming cream and fill the hot dish. Give them a chance to cook until nearly done and add a few pepperoni cuts to the other side. 3. Sprinkle mozzarella cheddar over the pepperoni alongside salt, pepper and basil and overlay the omelette over. 4. Let cook for one more moment and present with a side of bacon!

DAY 3 LUNCH

Lunch (makes 2 servings) Quick Asian Crack Slaw

Ingredients • 1 table spoon sesame seed oil (discretionary) • 1 clove garlic • ½ lb ground hamburger (we utilized 80% lean) • 5 oz. coleslaw plate of mixed greens blend • 1 table spoon olive oil • 1 table spoon soy sauce • Salt, pepper • 1 table spoon sesame seeds • 1 stalk green onion

Guidelines

1. Start by warming the sesame seed oil in a huge wok and pounding the garlic clove into it. Cook until fragrant. 2. Include the ground meat and say a final farewell to a wooden spoon. 3. When the ground meat is sautéed, around 5-10 minutes, include the coleslaw serving of mixed greens blend and hurl to consolidate. 4. Include olive oil and soy sauce. Mix and let cook for around 5 minutes for the coleslaw blend to wither. 5. Season with salt, pepper and sesame seeds. Present with a sprinkle of green onion and appreciate! 6. Sustenance is for 1/2 of the formula.

DAY 3 DINNER

Shrimp and Mushroom Zoodles

Ingredients • 1 tablespoon of olive oil • 8 oz. white mushrooms, cut • 1 table spoon butter • 6 oz. enormous shrimp, stripped • 1 huge zucchini • ¼ cup marinara sauce • Salt, pepper • 2 table spoon Parmesan cheddar

Guidelines 1. Heat the olive oil in an enormous skillet over medium warmth. 2. Fry the mushrooms until they've absorbed the vast majority of the oil. 3. Include spread and let the mushrooms cook until they've turned brilliant. 4. Include the shrimp and let them cook for around 5 minutes on both side. 5. When the shrimp are cooked and pink, hurl the zoodles in for around 2 minutes. 7. At that point, include the marinara sauce and season with salt and pepper. 8. Appreciate with a sprinkle of Parmesan

DAY 4 BREAKFAST

Velvety Scrambled Eggs

Ingredients • 4 enormous eggs • 2 table spoon spread • 4 strips bacon • 2 table spoon sharp cream • ½ table spoon salt • ¼ table spoon dark pepper • 1 stalk green onion

Guidelines

1. Break eggs and add the spread to a dish on medium-high heat. Blend continuously with a silicone spatula. 2. While mixing the eggs, let some bacon strips cook in another dish (or prepare them). 3. Interchange blending the eggs on the warmth and of the heat in 30-second interims. When they're nearly done, turn the warmth off. The eggs will keep cooking somewhat more from the remaining warmth from the container. 4. Include a tablespoon of harsh cream and season with salt and pepper. 5. Trimming with slashed green onion and appreciate!

DAY 4 LUNCH

Fast Asian Crack Slaw

Ingredients • 1 table spoon sesame seed oil (discretionary) • 1 clove garlic • ½ lb ground meat (we utilized 80% lean) • 5 oz. coleslaw serving of mixed greens blend • 1 table spoon olive oil • 1 table spoon soy sauce • Salt, pepper • 1 table spoon sesame seeds • 1 stalk green onion

Guidelines 1. Start by warming the sesame seed oil in a huge wok and squashing the garlic clove into it. Cook until fragrant. 2. Include the ground hamburger and say a final farewell to a wooden spoon. 3. When the ground hamburger is sautéed, around 5-10 minutes, include the coleslaw serving of mixed greens blend and hurl to consolidate. 4. Include olive oil and soy sauce. Blend and let cook for around 5 minutes for the coleslaw blend to shrink. 5. Season with salt, pepper and sesame seeds. Present with a sprinkle of green onion and appreciate! 6. Nourishment is for 1/2 of the formula.

DAY 4 DINNER

Low Carb Chicken Quesadilla

Ingredients • 1 low carb wrap • 3oz. Pepper jack cheddar destroyed • 2.5oz. chicken breast, grilled, crushed • ½ avocado, sliced dainty • 1 table spoon chopped jalapeño • ¼ table spoon salt

Directions

1. Spot the wrap on a skillet wide enough to allow the wrap to lay as completely level as conceivable on medium warmth. 2. Following 2 minutes, flip the fold around and start spreading out the pepper jack. Try not to get excessively near the corners (leave somewhat less than in inch from the edges of the wrap). 3. Include the chicken bosom, avocado and jalapeño to one portion of the wrap. 4. Overlap the fold around with a spatula and press down to smooth (not all that much!). This will guarantee the dissolved cheddar sticks the quesadilla together.

5. Remove the container and cut into thirds. Appreciate with salsa as well as acrid cream!

DAY 5 BREAKFAST

Green Breakfast Smoothie

Spices • 1.5 cups of almond milk • 1 oz. spinach • 50 grams avocado • 1 table spoon coconut oil • 10 drops fluid stevia • 1 scoop vanilla protein powder (around 30 grams)

Guidelines 1. Join all the smoothie ingredients in a blender or Nutribullet. 2. Mix on high until everything is smooth and velvety. 3. Appreciate

DAY 5 LUNCH

Ham and Cheddar Wraps

Ingredients • 1 low carb wrap • 2 table spoon mayonnaise • 2 oz. Cheddar, destroyed • 2 oz. store ham • Pickles or jalapenos to taste • Salt, pepper

Guidelines 1. Onto a low carb wrap, spread the mayonnaise. 2. Include the destroyed cheddar and ham cuts. 3. If you need, including a few pickles or jalapenos for something crisp and tasty. 4. Wrap it up tight and slice it to accommodate your lunch pack or appreciate immediately

DAY 5 DINNER

Avocado Lime Salmon and Cauli-rice

Ingredients • 50 grams cauliflower • ½ avocado • ½ lime • 1 table spoon red onion, diced • 1 6-oz. salmon filet (or chicken thighs) • Salt, pepper

Guidelines 1. Rice the cauliflower by beating it in a nourishment processor until it's rice. Cook it in a softly oiled search for gold 8 minutes. 2. In a nourishment processor, mix the avocado, the juice of 1/2 a lime and diced red onion until smooth and creamy. 3. Warmth a skillet with some oil and cook the salmon filet skin-side down for around 4-5 minutes. Season with salt and pepper while it's cooking. Flip the salmon and keep on cooking for an extra 4-5 minutes. (You can likewise set up some chicken thighs on the off chance that you don't care for salmon.) 5. When it's cooked, serve it over a bed of the cauliflower rice and a liberal touch of the avocado lime sauce.

DAY 6 BREAKFAST

Simple Blender Pancakes

Ingredients • 2 oz. cream cheddar • 2 enormous eggs • 1 scoop vanilla protein powder (around 30 grams) • 1 run cinnamon • 10 drops fluid stevia (discretionary) • 1 squeeze salt

Guidelines

1. Include every one of the ingredients into a blender or Nutribullet. 2. Mix on high until everything is smooth and creamy. 3. Warmth a frying pan to medium warmth and include the flapjack hitter into 4-5 inch distance across rounds. 4. Cook until you see air pockets shaping at the surface and the edges look dry. 5. Flip and then cook for

some more seconds. 6. Appreciate with spread and a sprinkle of sugar free maple syrup.

DAY 6 LUNCH

Fish Avocado Salad

Ingredients • 4 oz. canned fish • ½ stalk celery, diced • ½ avocado • 2 table spoon mayonnaise • 1 table spoon mustard • ½ table spoon new lemon juice • Salt, pepper • 1 hard-bubbled egg, stripped, slashed

Directions

1. Join the fish, celery and avocado. 2. Include mayo, mustard, lemon squeeze and flavours. 3. Add the egg to the fish serving of mixed greens. 4. Blend very well until every one of the ingredients is all around joined. 5. Pack it up and spare it for lunch!

DAY 6 DINNER

Mustard Lemon Pork and Green Beans

Ingredients • 2 4-oz. pork flanks • 1 table spoon olive oil • 1 cup green beans • Mustard Sauce • ¼ cup chicken soup • 2 table spoon overwhelming cream • ½ table spoon apple juice vinegar • ¼ lemon • ½ table spoon mustard

Guidelines

1. Pat pork midsections dry with a paper towel and season with salt and pepper.

2. On an enormous container with olive oil on high heat, singe the pork on the two sides for 2 minutes. 3. Put them

in a safe spot and deglaze the skillet with chicken juices, apple juice vinegar and substantial cream. Let this go to a stew. 4. Include the lemon juice, mustard and mix to join. Add pork midsections back to the skillet and flip once to cover them in the sauce. 5. Give them a chance to cook for 10 minutes with the top of the container left somewhat open. 6. Meal greens beans in a 350°F broiler for 10 minutes and serve together with sauce on top.

DAY 7 BREAKFAST

Wiener, Egg and Cheese

Ingredients • 3 oz. breakfast sausage (for example Jimmy Dean) • 1 enormous egg • 1 table spoon olive oil • 1 cut cheddar • Chives or green onion for enhancement

Guidelines

1. Cook the breakfast frankfurter and egg (just right or over simple) in a delicately oiled container. 2. Orchestrate them with a cut of cheddar and shower with some hot sauce on the off chance that you'd like. 3. Top with chives or green onion for topping.

DAY 7 LUNCH

Simple Cobb Salad

Ingredients • 1 huge hard-bubbled egg • 4 oz. chicken bosom • 1 cup spinach • 2 strips bacon • ¼ avocado • 1 table spoon olive oil • ½ table spoon white vinegar

Directions

1. Carry a pot of water to bubble and cook the egg for 10 minutes. When it's cooked, cool it in virus water and hack

it up. 2. On a grill, cook 4 oz. of chicken bosom and bacon to wanted freshness. 3. Generally, hack or tear spinach leaves and include the bacon, chicken and slashed egg. 4. Toss fifty-fifty an avocado and blend to split it up. 5. Dress with olive oil and vinegar or utilize a low carb Bleu cheddar dressing.

DAY 7 DINNER

Sriracha Lime Flank Steak

Ingredients • 7 oz. asparagus • 8 oz. flank steak • Salt, pepper • Sriracha Lime Sauce • ½ lime • 1 table spoon sriracha • ½ table spoon vinegar • Salt, pepper • 1 table spoon olive oil

Directions

1. Trim the closures off the asparagus and let them fry on medium warmth for around 10 minutes, hurling once in a while. 2. Carefuly seasoned the steak with salt and pepper. Sear for 5 minutes on each side for medium-uncommon. Include 1 moment each side for medium and 2 minutes for well-done. 3. Spread the steak and let rest for 5 minutes. In the meantime, crush crisp lime in a bowl and blend with sriracha, vinegar, salt and pepper. While whisking these together, slowly pour in olive oil to make an emulsion and thicken the sauce. 4. Cut steak slim and present with sauce and the asparagus.

CHAPTER 5- KETO FOR WOMEN RECIPES

Chocolate and Nutty Smoothies

Prep. Time: 5 minutes / Cook time: 5 minutes / Serves 2

1 tbsp. Nutella 1 banana

½ cup Milk 2 oz. Walnuts

1. Cut the banana into slices, add a cup of milk and a tablespoon of chocolate paste and walnuts (6–8 pieces).

2. For 1–2 minutes, ready to smooth with chocolate chips.

* Nutella can be replaced with half a melted chocolate bar. From nuts, you can use hazelnuts.

Calories: 351. Fat: 23 g. Protein: 8 g. Carbs: 33

BREAKFAST

Keto Taco

Prep. time: 10 minutes / Cook time: 20 minutes / Serves 3

Want to start the day unusual? Morning keto is such an amazing start to a beautiful day. Light and wonderful with a lot of bright colors and emotions.

8 oz. Mozzarella cheese, shredded; 6 Eggs, large 2 tbsp. Butter

3 Bacon stripes ½ Avocado 1 oz. Cheddar cheese, shredded Pepper and salt to taste

1. Heat an oven to 375 °F. Put the foil on a baking sheet and spread the bacon on it. Cook it for 15-20 minutes.
2. While bacon is cooked, put 3 oz. of mozzarella in a clean pan and cook cheese over medium heat.
3. Wait for the cheese to roast around the edges (about 2-3 minutes).
4. Use a pair of tongs and a wooden spoon to make a cheese shell for tacos.
5. Do the same with the rest of your cheese.
6. Cook the eggs in the oil, stirring occasionally. Season with salt and pepper.
7. Place a third of the eggs, avocado and bacon in each hardened taco casing.
8. Sprinkle with cheddar cheese. Add hot sauce and cilantro if desired.

Calories: 444. Fat: 36 g. Protein: 26 g. Carbs: 2.3

Keto Omelet with Goat Cheese and Spinach

Prep. time: 5 minutes / Cook time: 10 minutes / Serves 1

3 Large eggs 1 Medium green onion 1 oz. Goat cheese ¼ Onion

2 tbsp. Butter 2 cups Spinach 2 tbsp. Heavy cream Salt and pepper to taste

1. Cut the onion into long strips and fry it in oil until caramelized. Add the spinach to the pan and fry a little.
2. Remove the vegetables from the pan. Mix 3 large eggs, cream, salt and pepper together.

3. Pour the egg mixture into the pan and cook on medium heat.
4. As soon as the edges of the omelet begin to fry, add a spoonful of spinach and onions to 1/2 omelet. Sprinkle with chopped goat cheese.
5. When the top of the omelet is ready, you can serve. If you like, decorate with onions on top.

Calories: 621. Fat: 55 g. Protein: 37 g. Carbs: 4.8

Chicken and Cheese Quesadilla

Prep. time: 10 minutes / Cook time: 15 minutes / Serves 4

For lozenges: 6 Eggs 4 oz. Coconut flour 6 oz. Heavy cream ½ tsp. Xanthan gum Pink salt and pepper 1 tbsp. Olive oil for frying

For the quesadilla: 4 oz. Cheddar cheese, shredded 8 oz. Chicken breast cooked and shredded 1 tbsp. Parsley, chopped (optional)

1. Mix in a bowl all the ingredients for the cakes, whisk well and let the dough stand for 8-10 minutes.
2. Heat the oil in a frying pan over medium heat and fry the tortillas for 2-3 minutes on each side or until cooked. Set aside to cool.
3. Heat a clean griddle over medium heat, put one tortilla, sprinkle with cheese, cover with a lid and wait until the cheese begins to melt. Then add chopped chicken meat, more cheese and cover with a second flat cake.

When the cheese has melted, remove the quesadilla from the pan, cut into four slices and sprinkle with fresh parsley before serving (optional).

NOTE: For best results, use ground coconut flour. This will help with the texture, and you can make thinner cakes. Xanthan gum will help make the tortilla strong and elastic. You can substitute fat cream with unsweetened almond milk. You can also reduce the number of eggs and add extra egg white. However, you will need to test and adjust the amount of flour used to obtain the desired consistency.

Calories: 382. Fat: 31 g. Protein: 23 g. Carbs: 2.3

Vegetarian Scramble

Prep. time: 5 minutes / Cook time: 15 minutes / Serves 5

The recipe is easy to prepare but tasty avocados, tomatoes and cheeses will lift your spirits and energize for great deeds.

1 lb. Tofu cheese 3 tbsp. Avocado oil 2 tbsp. Chopped onion 1½ tbsp. Food yeast ½ tsp. Garlic powder

½ tsp. Turmeric ½ tsp. Salt 1 cup Spinach 3 Grape tomatoes 3 oz. Vegan Cheddar Cheese

1. Wrap the tofu in several layers of paper or cloth towels, and gently squeeze some water. Put aside.
2. In a skillet over medium heat, fry the chopped onion in 1/3 tbsp. Avocado butter until onion is soft and translucent.
3. Place the tofu in the pan and stir well with a fork.

4. Pour the remaining oil and sprinkle with dry seasoning.
5. Fry the tofu over medium heat, stirring occasionally until most of the liquid has evaporated.
6. Add the spinach, dice the tomatoes and cheddar cheese, and cook for a minute or until the spinach has faded and the cheese has melted.
7. Serve hot and store leftovers in the refrigerator for a maximum of three days.

Calories: 211. Fat: 17.6 g. Protein: 10 g. Carbs: 4.7

Burger with Guacamole and Egg

Prep. Time: 5 minutes / Cook time: 10 minutes / Serves 1

Sometimes in the morning you really want a juicy burger with various spices. Therefore, I have prepared for you this wonderful recipe. Juicy meat, cheerful guacamole, an egg and 10 minutes is all you need to enjoy your favorite keto burgher. Everyone around will want the same.

5 oz. Ground beef 4 Bacon, slices 3 oz. Guacamole 1 Egg

1 tbsp. Olive oil (for frying) ½ tsp. Italian seasoning Salt and pepper to taste

1. In a small bowl, mix ground beef with Italian seasoning, salt and pepper. Form a small patty.
2. Put on a cutting board 4 strips of bacon crosswise, cutlet on top, and then wrap bacon around it.
3. Heat 1/2 tablespoons of olive oil in a frying pan over medium heat, add the cutlet in bacon and fry

3 minutes (or more, depending on thickness) on each side.
4. Add the remaining 1/2 tablespoons of oil to the pan and fry the egg, with the liquid yolk inside.
5. Put a guacamole, a fried egg on a cutlet, and, if necessary, season with salt and pepper. Cut in half and serve immediately.

Calories: 443. Fat: 33 g. Protein: 32.5 g. Carbs: 2.4

Stuffed Avocado

Prep. time: 5 minutes / Cook time: 10 minutes / Serves 1

1 Avocado, pitted and cut in half 1 tbsp. Butter, salted 3 Large eggs

3 slices of bacon, cut into small pieces Salt and black pepper, to taste

1. Clean out most of the avocado pulp, leaving about 1.5 cm around.
2. Place a large frying pan over low heat and add butter. While the butter is melting, break the eggs into a bowl and whisk them, adding a pinch of salt and pepper.
3. Place bacon on one side of the pan and fry for a couple of minutes. On the other side pour the egg mixture and stir them regularly.
4. Eggs and bacon should be prepared 5 minutes after adding eggs to the pan. If you find that the eggs are cooked a little before the bacon, remove the scrambled eggs and place them in a bowl.
5. Mix the bacon and scrambled eggs together, and then fill the avocado halves with the mixture.

PER SERVING Calories: 500. Fat: 40 g. Protein: 25 g. Carbs: 11

Omelet with Mushrooms and Goat Cheese

Prep. time: 5 minutes / Cook time: 10 minutes / Serves 1

3 Large eggs 2 tsp. Heavy cream 3 oz. Chopped mushrooms 1 tsp. Olive oil

2 oz. Crumbled goat cheese Seasoning to taste Green onions for garnish

1. Heat olive oil in a pan. Fry the mushrooms until soft, about. 4 minutes.
2. While the mushrooms are cooking, beat the eggs with heavy cream and a small amount of seasoning.
3. Pour the egg mixture over the mushrooms and cook for about 2-3 minutes.
4. Add goat cheese. Fold the omelet in half and continue cooking until the cheese starts to melt.
5. Serve with spring onions or another side dish to your taste.

Calories: 515. Fat: 39.5 g. Protein: 21 g. Carbs: 4.2

Fat Bombs

Neapolitan Fatty Bombs

Prep. time: 10 minutes / Cook time: 15 minutes / Serves 24

½ cup Butter ½ cup Coconut oil ½ cup Sour cream ½ cup Cream cheese 2 tbsp. Erythritol

25 drops Liquid stevia 2 tbsp. Cocoa powder 1 tsp. Vanilla extract 2 medium strawberries

1. Using a blender, mix all the ingredients (except cocoa powder, vanilla and strawberry) in a bowl.
2. Divide the mixture between 3 bowls. Add cocoa powder to one, vanilla to another, and strawberries to third.
3. Pour the chocolate mixture into the mold and place in the freezer for 30 minutes. Repeat the process with vanilla and strawberry layers.
4. Now put all freeze for at least 1 hour.

Calories: 102. Fat: 11 g. Protein: 1 g. Carbs: 0.5

Chocolate-Coconut Fat Bombs with Almonds

Prep. time: 5 minutes / Cook time: 15 minutes / Serves 12

1 cup Coconut chips 3 tbsp. Fat coconut milk 3 tbsp. Coconut oil (melted) ½ tsp. Vanilla extract

4 oz. Chocolate chips, no sugar A pinch of salt 2 oz. Keto-friendly sweetener 24 Almond, pieces

1. Put 2 tablespoons of melted coconut oil, coconut milk, sweetener, coconut chips, vanilla extract and salt in a small bowl.
2. Divide the mixture into 12 servings and place them on a baking sheet with parchment paper. Put in the freezer for 5 minutes, then put on each fat bomb 1-2 things almonds.
3. Melt the chocolate chips together with 2 teaspoons of coconut oil in the microwave.

4. Remove the bombs from the freezer, pour each of the chocolate mixture and cool.

Calories: 92. Fat: 9 g. Protein: 2 g. Carbs: 1.5

Spicy Fat Bombs

Prep. time: 5 minutes / Cook time: 15 minutes / Serves 12

6 MCT powder, scoops 10 Liquid stevia, drops 1 tsp. Turmeric 1 tbsp. Black sesame seeds

Pinch Chinese 5 Spice Blend A pinch of black pepper ½ tsp. Cinnamon 2½ fl. oz. Warm water

1. Mix all the dry ingredients in a small bowl.
2. Add warm water and mix until smooth.
3. Spread the mixture evenly over 12 silicone molds, about 1 tbsp. 1 on each.
4. Put in the fridge so that the fat bombs are well frozen. Always keep them frozen, otherwise they will quickly melt.

Calories: 81. Fat: 8 g. Protein: 1 g. Carbs: 1.5

Coffee Fat Bombs

Prep. time: 5 minutes / Cook time: 30 minutes / Serves 12

4 oz. Butter 2 oz. Ghee butter (melted) 2 oz. Heavy cream 1 tbsp. Milk to your taste Double espresso

2 oz. Keto-friendly sweetener of your choice 1 tsp. Vanilla extract A pinch of salt

1. Add all ingredients to a small food processor and whip at high speed until airy.
2. Add sweetener to taste to taste.
3. Pour into molds and refrigerate for 30 minutes (or more if you wish)

Calories: 61. Fat: 5 g. Protein: 1 g. Carbs: 1

Almond Coconut Fat Bombs

Prep. time: 5 minutes / Cook time: 20 minutes / Serves 10

2 fl. oz. Almond oil 2 fl. oz Coconut oil

2 tbsp. Cocoa powder 2 fl. oz Erythritol, to your taste

1. Mix almond and coconut oil in a microwave dish.
2. Heat the mixture in the microwave for 30-45 seconds and mix until a homogeneous mass. Add erythritol and cocoa powder, and mix to complete the mix.
3. Pour the mass into mini cupcake molds and refrigerate in the refrigerator.

Calories: 89. Fat: 9.3 g. Protein: 1.5 g. Carbs: 1

Pumpkin Fat Spice Bombs

Prep. time: 5 minutes / Cook time: 10 minutes / Serves 9

8 oz. Raw cashews 4 oz. Raw macadamia nuts 4 oz. Coconut chips 3 fl. oz. Pumpkin puree

2 tbsp. MCT oils 2 tsp. Cinnamon, ground 2 tsp. Ginger, ground Neutral oil (avocado oil)

1. Put all the ingredients in a food processor and mix to form a dough.
2. Lightly grease your hands with neutral oil, such as avocado oil. Using a spoon, take about 3.5 -4 oz. of the batter into lightly oiled hands and form a ball. Postpone and repeat the process (about 9 "bombs" in total).
3. Decorate fat bombs with savory coconut chips.
4. Such fatty bombs can be eaten immediately, or stored in a refrigerator / freezer.

Calories: 217. Fat: 19 g. Protein: 5 g. Carbs: 5

Cheese Fat Bombs in Bacon

Prep. time: 5 minutes / Cook time: 20 minutes / Serves 20

8 oz. Mozzarella cheese 4 tbsp. Almond flour 4 tbsp. Butter, melted 3 tbsp. Psyllium powder 1 Egg Salt, to taste

1 tsp. Black pepper 1/8 tsp. Garlic powder 1/8 tsp. Onion powder 20 Bacon, slices 1 cup oil or lard (for frying)

1. Microwave half the cheese for 45-60 seconds or until it melts and becomes sticky.
2. Heat the butter in the microwave for 15-20 seconds until completely melted, then mix it with cheese and egg.
3. Add psyllium husks, almond flour and spices. Mix again and lay out the dough rectangle.
4. Fill the rectangle with the rest of the cheese and fold it in half (horizontally), then in half (vertically).
5. Trim the edges and form into a rectangle. Cut 20 square pieces.

6. Wrap each piece of dough with a piece of bacon, using toothpicks to fasten it.
7. Put each piece in boiling oil and cook for 1-3 minutes.

Calories: 93. Fat: 8 g. Protein: 5 g. Carbs: 1

Salads

Vegetable Salad with Bacon and Cheese

Prep. time: 5 minutes / Cook time: 10 minutes / Serves 6

4 oz. Lettuce 3 oz. Spinach 2 oz. Curly cabbage 6 slices of cooked bacon 12 pcs. grape tomato

1. 1 Avocado, peeled and sliced 2 oz. Blue cheese 3 tbsp. Sour cream 2 ½ tbsp. Mayonnaise
2. In a small bowl, mix the sour cream and mayonnaise.
3. Mix with half the blue cheese and set aside.
4. In a large salad bowl, mix the remaining ingredients.
5. Spread the salad into portions and place the blue cheese dressing on top.

Calories: 183. Fat: 16 g. Protein: 6.5 g. Carbs: 2.5

Salad with Chicken Breast and Greens

Prep. time: 10 minutes / Cook time: 30 minutes / Serves 2

2 tbsp. Pesto sauce 2 fl. oz. Balsamic vinegar 1 tsp. Olive oil 6 oz. Chicken breast 4 cup Spring greens

1 oz. Fresh mozzarella ¼ Avocado, diced 6 Cherry tomatoes 1 tbsp. Fresh basil for decoration

1. Prepare the marinade by mixing pesto, balsamic vinegar and olive oil.
2. Set aside a portion of the marinade for the salad, and pour the remaining chicken breast. Refrigerate marinate for at least 20 minutes.
3. Take the salad. Start with greens, then layered with fresh mozzarella, avocado and tomatoes.
4. Once the chicken is pickled, heat the medium-sized griddle, and then add a little olive oil.
5. Fry each side of the breast for 7-10 minutes.
6. Slice the chicken breast and place on the previously prepared salad.
7. Pour the remaining balsamic pesto and add some chopped fresh basil.

Calories: 306. Fat: 16 g. Protein: 25 g. Carbs: 6.5

Salmon Salad

Prep. time: 5 minutes / Cook time: 10 minutes / Serves 2

2 Sheets of lettuce 6 leaves, Fresh basil, finely chopped ½ tsp. Garlic powder 1 tsp. Lemon juice

4 tbsp. Mayonnaise 5 oz. Salmon 1 oz. Red onion, chopped ½ Avocado, diced 2 tbsp. Parmesan cheese, diced

1. Rinse well and clean the lettuce leaves - they will serve as plates.
2. Mix lemon juice, chopped basil and garlic powder.

3. Add mayonnaise and mix well. Set aside.
4. Fill each "plate" of lettuce with half of the finely chopped salmon, and then avocado and onion rings.
5. Top with evenly arrange the mayonnaise (earlier about 2 tablespoons per serving), then place the parmesan cubes.

Calories: 373. Fat: 31 g. Protein: 19.6 g. Carbs: 2.5

Simple Cabbage and Egg Keto Salad

Prep. time: 10 minutes / Cook time: 10 minutes / Serves 6

1 lb. Cauliflower flowers 4 oz. Keto mayonnaise 1 tsp. Yellow mustard 1½ tsp. Fresh dill Ground black pepper and salt, to taste 2 oz. Finely chopped dill

1 Celery stalk, finely chopped 2 oz. Red onion, chopped 1 tbsp. Salted keto cucumber, chopped 6 Hard-boiled eggs, chopped Paprika, for garnish

1. Pour some water (about 2.5 cm) into a large saucepan, put 1 tsp. of salt and bring to a boil. Add cauliflower and cook until ready, from 8 to 10 minutes. Drain and set aside in a large bowl.
2. In a small bowl, mix mayonnaise, mustard, dill, a pinch of salt and pepper. Set aside.
3. Crush 4 eggs and add to the cauliflower bowl. Slice the remaining two eggs.
4. Add pickled cucumber, celery, 1/4 teaspoon salt, pepper and red onion. Add all the ingredients to the cauliflower and shake gently.

5. Garnish with the remaining chopped eggs and sprinkle with paprika.

Calories: 222. Fat: 20 g. Protein: 8 g. Carbs: 2

Light Pea and Green Onion Salad

Prep. time: 5 minutes / Cook time: 10 minutes / Serves

2 oz. Pea 2 tsp. Green onions ½ tsp. Soy sauce 2 tsp. Olive oil

½ tsp. Apple vinegar ½ tsp. Sesame oil ½ tsp. Sesame seeds Garlic powder, to taste

1. Slice the green onions and peas diagonally.
2. Mix the chopped vegetables with the remaining ingredients and mix. Cover and refrigerate for 2 hours.
3. Serve with the main course of your choice - grilled chicken, shrimps, salmon, etc.

Calories: 136. Fat: 14 g. Protein: 2.5 g. Carbs: 3

Keto-Salsa with Avocado and Shrimps

Prep. time: 10 minutes / Cook time: 10 minutes / Serves 4

8 oz. Peeled raw shrimp 1 tbsp. Olive oil 1 Lemon (juice) 1 Avocado, diced 1 Tomato, diced

1 Cucumber, diced 1/4 Onion, diced 2 oz. Cilantro, chopped Salt and black pepper, to taste

1. Season the shrimp with salt and pepper. Put the pan on a medium-high heat and pour olive oil. Once the oil has warmed up, add the shrimp and

fry one side for 2-3 minutes, then turn to the other.
2. Remove the shrimps from the pan and put them on a cutting board. Slice and transfer to a large bowl.
3. Squeeze the marinade lemon juice into the bowl. Mix well and let stand for a while.
4. Add pieces of avocado, tomatoes and cucumbers to the bowl.
5. Mix with chopped onion and cilantro. Mix well all together.

Calories: 283. Fat: 18.8 g. Protein: 18 g. Carbs: 6.2

Keto Salad Taco

Prep. time: 10 minutes / Cook time: 20 minutes / Serves 4

1 lb. Ground beef from grass-fed meat 1 tsp. Ground cumin ½ tsp. Chili powder 1 tbsp. Garlic powder ½ tbsp. Paprika Salt and pepper, to taste 4 cup Roman lettuce

1 Tomato 4 oz. Cheddar cheese 4 oz. Cilantro 1 Avocado 4 oz. Favorite salsa 2 small limes 1 cup Cucumber, sliced

1. Heat a large skillet over medium heat and pour in some coconut oil. Add ground beef and all seasonings.
2. Mix well and fry until brown. Remove from heat and cool slightly.
3. Mix roman lettuce, vegetables, cheese and chopped avocado. Top with meat, salsa and a generous portion of lime juice. Mix everything well.

Calories: 430. Fat: 31 g. Protein: 29 g. Carbs:

Snacks

Quick Keto Bread

Prep. time: 5 minutes / Cook time: 10 minutes / Serves 10

2 tbsp. Almond flour ½ tbsp. Coconut flour 1/4 tsp. Baking powder 1 Egg

½ tbsp. Ghee or butter 1 tbsp. Unsweetened milk of your choic

1. Mix all ingredients in a small bowl and whisk until smooth.
2. Grease a glass bowl or microwave dish with butter, ghee or coconut oil.
3. Pour the dough into a mold and place in the microwave at high temperature for 90 seconds.
4. Slice and pour melted butter as desired.

Calories: 45. Fat: 20 g. Protein: 7 g. Carbs: 3

Note: If you do not have a microwave, try frying the dough in a small amount of butter / coconut oil or ghee. The same cooking time, the same easy recipe is just a slightly different texture.

Energy Keto Bars with Nuts and Seeds

Prep. time: 10 minutes / Cook time: 25 minutes / Serves 8

2 tbsp. Butter or coconut oil 2 fl. oz. Sugar-free 1 tsp. Vanilla extract 8 oz. Almond, chopped 8 oz. Raw macadamia nuts (finely chopped) 4 oz. Pumpkin seed

2 tbsp. Hemp seed 1-2 tsp. Keto sweetener (if necessary) 4 oz. Low sugar chocolate chips ½ tsp. Coconut or butter, or ghee oil

1. Preheat the oven to 350 °F degrees and lay out a baking dish with parchment paper. Put all the nuts and seeds in a large bowl, and mix.
2. Melt butter or coconut oil with vanilla extract and syrup in a small saucepan over low heat.
3. Pour the hot mixture over the nuts and seeds, and shake well. If necessary, add keto sweetener (erythritol, stevia, etc.)
4. Pour the resulting mass into the prepared baking dish.
5. Bake for about 22-25 minutes until the top turns golden brown. Allow the mixture to cool for at least 45 minutes.
6. Melt the chocolate and 1/2 tsp of coconut oil in the microwave or on the stove. Pour a mixture of baked nuts and seeds.
7. Put in the freezer for 10-15 minutes. Remove from the mold and cut into 8 pieces.

Calories: 303. Fat: 29 g. Protein: 8 g. Carbs: 4

Low-Carb Flax Bread

Prep. time: 10 minutes / Cook time: 15 minutes / Serves 8

1 oz. Almond flour 1½ Flaxseed 1 tsp. Baking powder Salt, to taste ½ tsp. Vinegar

4 drops Liquid stevia 3 oz. Raw whisked egg 1 fl. oz. Coconut oil or butter (melted)

1. Mix together all the dry ingredients, then mix the wet ones.
2. Stir dry ingredients with wet ones.
3. Spread the dough into a lightly oiled form.
4. Bake at 350 °F degrees for 8–10 minutes.

Calories: 35. Fat: 42 g. Protein: 14 g. Carbs: 6

Keto Mini Pizza

Prep. time: 5 minutes / Cook time: 15 minutes / Serves 4

1 oz. Keto mayonnaise 1 tbsp. Raw eggs 2 tsp. Coconut oil, melted 2 tsp. Almond flour

1 tsp. Coconut flour ½ tsp. Psyllium powder A pinch of baking powder and baking soda

1. Heat the oven to 400 °F degrees.
2. Mix all the ingredients well to form a dough. Make sure there are no lumps in it.
3. Leave the dough to stand for about 5 minutes.
4. Divide the dough into 3-4 small balls, about 2.5 cm in diameter.
5. Lay out a baking sheet with parchment paper. Put dough balls on the parchment and press down on them to make small pizzas.
6. Put the stuffing on the raw dough and bake for 7-9 minutes.

Calories: 112. Fat: 28 g. Protein: 4 g. Carbs: 2

Baked Eggs with Ham and Asparagus

Prep. time: 5 minutes / Cook time: 15 minutes / Serves

6 Eggs 6 slices (about 4 oz.) Italian ham 8 oz. Asparagus

A few sprigs of fresh marjoram 1 tbsp. Butter or ghee

1. Heat the oven to 350 °F degrees.
2. Grease a muffin tray.
3. Lay the ham down and around the hole so as to cover the bottom and sides.
4. Add a few twigs of marjoram.
5. Pour 1 egg into each form.
6. Put in the oven and bake 10 - 12 minutes until cooked.
7. Pull out and allow to cool for a few minutes.
8. Steam the asparagus, then season it with butter.
9. Put all the ingredients on a plate and enjoy.

Calories: 424. Fat: 33 g. Protein: 30 g. Carbs: 2.5

Eggplant Keto Chips

Prep. time: 5 minutes / Cook time: 20 minutes / Serves 4

2 fl. oz. Olive oil 1 Large eggplant (thinly sliced) Sal and pepper to taste 1 tsp. Garlic powder

½ tsp. Dry basil ½ tsp. Dried oregano 2 tbsp. Parmesan cheese

1. Preheat oven to 350 °F degrees.
2. Add 1/4 cup olive oil and dried spices to a small bowl. Roll the sliced eggplant in oil and spices, and place it on a baking sheet.

3. Bake for about 15-20 minutes, until the chips are evenly fried. Turn them over a couple of times during cooking.
4. Remove from the oven and sprinkle with Parmesan cheese (optional)

Calories: 60. Fat: 5 g. Protein: 2 g. Carbs: 1

Cheese Keto Sticks

Prep. time: 5 minutes / Cook time: 15 minutes / Serves 3

3 Mozzarella cheese sticks (cut in half) 4 oz. Almond flour 1 tbsp. Italian seasoning mixes 2 tbsp. Grated parmesan cheese

1 Big egg Salt, to taste 2 tbsp. Coconut oil 1 tbsp. Chopped parsley

1. Put the cheese in the freezer overnight so that it hardens.
2. Then add coconut oil to a medium sized cast iron skillet and heat it over low to medium heat.
3. Break the egg into a shallow bowl and whisk well. In a separate bowl, mix the almond flour, parmesan cheese and seasonings.
4. Roll cheese sticks in an egg, then dry breading. Put on a wire rack and bake until golden brown on all sides for about 12 minutes.
5. Place chopsticks on paper towels to soak up the oil.
6. Serve with low-carb marinara sauce and parsley (optional).

Calories: 436. Fat: 39 g. Protein: 20 g. Carbs: 5

LUNCH

Chicken Keto Nuggets

Prep. time: 15 minutes / Cook time: 6 hours / Serves 4

1 oz. Whipped egg whites 1 oz. Chicken breast cooked and minced ½ oz. Coconut flour ½ tsp. Baking powder

1 fl. oz. Olive oil ½ oz. Melted butter 1 oz. Fatty 40% cream Salt, pepper, a pinch of garlic powder, optional

1. Mix shredded chicken with coconut flour, baking powder and seasoning. The mixture should look very dry.
2. Add butter and mix again. Add whipped egg whites and mix until smooth.
3. Pour olive oil into a small non-stick pan. Spread the chicken-egg mixture in small pieces and fry for about 1 minute on each side.
4. Serve with whipped cream, diluted with water, like "milk".

Calories: 136. Fat: 41 g. Protein: 9 g. Carbs: 2

Champignon Keto Burger

Prep. time: 5 minutes / Cook time: 15 minutes / Serves 4

2 Large champignons, without legs 2 tbsp. Olive oil 1 tbsp. Balsamic vinegar 2 Slices of bacon 4 oz. Ground beef ½ tsp. Garlic powder

½ tsp. Onion powder ½ tsp. Worcestershire Sauce 1 Cheddar cheese, slice 1 Slice of tomato 2 oz. Mixed greens or arugula 1 tbsp. Low-sugar ketchup

1. Put the mushroom caps in a bowl or shallow plate, and add olive oil, balsamic vinegar and half the salt and pepper; marinate for at least 30 minutes.
2. Cook the bacon in a frying pan over medium heat until crisp, turning a couple of times to fry each side evenly. Set aside.
3. Preheat the oven and turn on the grill function (270 °F degrees). Mix in a bowl ground beef, garlic and onion powder, Worcestershire sauce, and the remaining salt and pepper. Form the patties for burgers.
4. Put the caps of champignons and cutlets on the grill, and cook for about 3-4 minutes on each side until they are soft. At the last minute, put the cheese on the cutlets so that it melts.
5. Assemble the hamburger with bacon and the rest of the stuffing between the mushroom caps.

Calories: 771. Fat: 67 g. Protein: 37 g. Carbs: 4

Nourishing Beef Soup

Prep. time: 10 minutes / Cook time: 30 minutes / Serves

1 lb. Ground beef 5 Slices of bacon 1 tbsp. Olive oil 1 tbsp. Minced garlic 1 cup Chopped celery 1½ cup Bone broth

1 cup Shredded cheddar 2 fl. oz. Fat whipped cream 2 tsp. Psyllium powder 4 oz. Shredded cheddar cheese ½ oz. Chopped green onions ½ cup Sour cream

1. Fry the bacon over medium heat, then place it on paper towels to remove excess fat. Then crush it into pieces.
2. Then fry the ground beef over medium heat. After cooking, drain the fat and transfer the minced meat to a bowl.
3. In the same pan, melt butter over medium heat. Add chopped garlic and fry until fragrant.
4. Add the celery and cook until slightly softened, about 5 minutes.
5. Put the ground beef in the pan. Add beef broth, cheddar, rich whipped cream, sautéed celery with garlic, bacon, salt and pepper. Cook for 20 minutes, stirring occasionally.
6. To obtain the desired thickness, add psyllium powder.
7. Pour into portions and add a side dish in the form of cheese, green onions and sour cream (optional).

Calories: 349. Fat: 27 g. Protein: 23 g. Carb

Keto Cheeseburger with Bacon

Prep. time: 10 minutes / Cook time: 30 minutes / Serves 2

For the dough: 8 oz. Mozzarella, shredded 4 oz. Almond flour 1 tbsp. Cream cheese

For filling: 5 oz. Ground beef 1 Slice of cheddar cheese, cut into quarters

1 tsp. Mustard 4 Bacon, slices 1 Whisked egg 1 tsp. Sesame 1 tsp. Olive oil Salad Leaves for Garnish (Optional)

1. Preheat oven to 420 °F degrees.
2. Mix mozzarella, almond flour and cream cheese in a bowl. Heat the mixture in the microwave for 1 minute, mix and re-set in the microwave for 1 minute.
3. Form two patties from ground beef. Put on the cutting board 4 strips of bacon crosswise, cutlet on top, then cheddar slices, the second cutlet, and then wrap all the bacon.
4. Heat the olive oil in a frying pan over medium heat, put the patties in bacon and fry for 3 minutes on each side.
5. Roll the dough between 2 sheets of parchment paper. Remove the top sheet and place mustard in the center of the dough. On top, put the patty in bacon and wrap the dough.
6. Put the burger in the oven, coat with beaten egg, sprinkle with sesame seeds and bake for 15-20 minutes or until golden brown.
7. Take out and serve with sheets of greens.

Calories: 411. Fat: 32 g. Protein: 27 g. Carbs: 3

Spicy Keto Soup with Mushrooms

Prep. time: 10 minutes / Cook time: 30 minutes / Serves 4

1 tbsp. Olive oil 1 Onion (thinly sliced) 1 tbsp. Fresh grated ginger 3 Garlic, cloves (finely chopped) 1 tsp. Chile 1 tbsp. Fish sauce

2 fl. oz. Soy sauce 2 fl. oz. Rice vinegar 4 oz. Mushrooms (thinly sliced) 4 Hard boiled eggs 2-3 packets of shirataki noodles 5 cup Bone broth

1. Pour oil into a large saucepan and put on medium heat. Add the onion and cook for 2-3 minutes until soft.
2. Add the remaining ingredients to the pan (except eggs and noodles). Cook over low heat for 20-30 minutes.
3. Remove the noodles from the package and rinse well under cold water.
4. Add seasoning to the broth and mix with noodles.
5. Pour the broth into portions. Add hard-boiled eggs, chopped chicken or beef, cilantro, sesame seeds, chopped green onions and chili sauce (all optional).

Calories: 103. Fat: 13 g. Protein: 12 g. Carbs: 7

Greek Keto Moussaka

Prep. time: 10 minutes / Cook time: 30 minutes / Serves

For filling: ½ Chopped eggplant 10 oz. Minced chicken 3 tbsp. Marinara sauce 1 Minced garlic ½ Chopped onion 1 tsp. Dried oregano 1 tsp. Paprika

½ tsp. Ground cinnamon 2 tbsp. Olive oil

For the sauce: 3 tbsp. Heavy cream 3 tbsp. Cream cheese 3 oz. Crushed cheddar cheese 1 Minced garlic

1. Lay out a foil baking sheet. Cut the eggplants, put them on a baking sheet and pour olive oil. Bake the eggplants for 5 minutes or until golden brown.
2. Heat olive oil in a frying pan, add chopped onion, chopped garlic and fry until soft. Add chopped chicken and seasonings, and fry until the meat is

cooked. Add the marinara sauce, mix and cook for another 3 minutes.
3. Mix half the crushed cheddar cheese, cream cheese, heavy cream, garlic and salt in a saucepan, and cook on low heat until the cheese is melted and the sauce becomes thick and uniform.
4. Preheat oven to 400 °F degrees. Place the pieces of fried eggplant on a baking sheet, top the chicken mixture, pour the sauce, sprinkle with the remaining cheese and bake for 20 minutes.
5. Let the dish stand for 5 minutes before serving. May be served with green salad or greens.

Calories: 358. Fat: 29 g. Protein: 20 g. Carbs: 4

Almond Pancakes with Shrimp and Cheese

Prep. time: 10 minutes / Cook time: 10 minutes / Serves 8

1 lb. Shrimp cooked and chopped 2 oz. Almond flour 1 Whisked egg 2 oz. Mozzarella, shredded

3 tbsp. Parmesan cheese, grated 1 tbsp. Fresh dill, chopped 1½ tbsp. Olive or coconut oil, for frying Salt and pepper, to taste

1. Mix the shrimp, egg, almond flour, cheese, dill and seasonings in a bowl and mix well until smooth.
2. Using a tablespoon to form pancakes. The size of each depends on your taste.
3. Heat the oil in a pan over medium heat and fry pancakes for 3-4 minutes on each side or until cooked.

4. Put on a plate and serve with herbs and aioli, or any other sauce of your choice.

Calories: 364. Fat: 21 g. Protein: 41 g. Carbs: 2

DINNER

Baked Halibut Cheese Breaded

Prep. time: 10 minutes / Cook time: 15 minutes / Serves 6

2 lb. Halibut (about 6 fillets) 1 tbsp. Butter 3 tbsp. Grated parmesan cheese 1 tbsp. Bread crumbs

2 tsp. Garlic powder 1 tbsp. Dried parsley Salt and pepper, to taste

1. Preheat the oven to 400 °F degrees. Mix all ingredients thoroughly in a bowl, except the plate.
2. Dry the fish fillets with a paper towel and place each piece on a greased buttered parchment tray.
3. Spread the cheese mixture into pieces of fish so that it covers its top.
4. Bake the fish for 10-12 minutes (turn the baking tray at least once).
5. Increase heat for 2–3 minutes until the top is golden brown. Check readiness with a fork.

Calories: 330. Fat: 30 g. Protein: 13 g. Carbs: 2

Tandoori Chicken Legs

Prep. time: 10 minutes / Cook time: 25 minutes / Serves 2

2 Whole chicken legs 4 fl. oz. Fatty Greek yogurt 2 tbsp. Olive oil ½ tsp. Cumin ½ tsp. Turmeric ½ tsp. Coriander 1/4 tsp. Cardamom

½ tsp. Cayenne pepper 1 tsp. Paprika Pinch of Nutmeg 1 Minced garlic clove ½ tsp. Fresh ginger 2 tbsp. Lime juice Salt and pepper, to taste

1. Heat olive oil in a small frying pan over medium heat. Add cumin, turmeric, coriander, cardamom, cayenne pepper, paprika and a pinch of nutmeg. Heat the spices, then remove from heat and cool.
2. Mix in a bowl yogurt with spiced oil, lime juice, ginger, chopped garlic, salt and pepper.
3. Make 3-4 deep cuts on each leg and pour spicy yogurt into them. Cover and refrigerate for 6 hours.
4. Lubricate the rack for frying olive oil and place on a baking sheet. Put the chicken on the rack and fry for 5 minutes on each side.
5. Set the oven to 360 °F degrees and continue cooking for 25 minutes.
6. Serve with cauliflower rice.

Calories: 372. Fat: 28 g. Protein: 30 g. Carbs: 2

Baked Eggplant with Cheese

Prep. time: 15 minutes / Cook time: 60 minutes / Serves 4

1 Large eggplant, sliced 1 Big egg ½ cup Parmesan cheese, grated ¼ cup Pork dough

½ tbsp. Italian seasoning 1 cup low-sugar tomato sauce ½ cup Mozzarella, shredded 4 tbsp. Butter

Instructions

1. Preheat oven to 400 °F degrees. Put the sliced eggplant on a baking sheet lined with a paper towel and sprinkle with salt on both sides. Let stand for at least 30 minutes so that all the water comes out of the eggplant.
2. Mix the chopped pork cracklings, parmesan cheese and Italian seasoning in a shallow dish. Set aside.
3. In a separate small plate, beat an egg.
4. Melt the butter and grease the baking dish with it.
5. Dip each piece of eggplant in a beaten egg, and then in a mixture of parmesan and cracklings, covering each side with crumbs.
6. Place the eggplants in a baking dish and bake for 20 minutes. Turn the eggplant slices over and bake for another 20 minutes or until golden brown.
7. Top with tomato sauce and sprinkle with chopped mozzarella.
8. Return the mold to the oven for another 5 minutes, or until the cheese has melted.

Calories: 376. Fat: 28 g. Protein: 19 g. Carbs: 7

Shrimp and Zucchini with Alfredo Sauce

Prep. time: 5 minutes / Cook time: 15 minutes / Serves 6

8 oz. Shrimp, peeled 2 tbsp. Butter ½ tsp Minced garlic 1 tbsp. Fresh lemon juice

2 Zucchini 2 oz. Heavy cream 3 oz. Parmesan cheese Salt and pepper to taste

1. Use the scoop to make zucchini noodles.
2. Heat the butter in a frying pan, add the chopped garlic, red pepper and fry for 1 minute, stirring constantly.
3. Add shrimp and simmer for about 3 minutes. Add salt and pepper, remove from pan and set aside.
4. In the same pan (with shrimp juice), add heavy cream, lemon juice, parmesan, and cook for 2 minutes.
5. Add the noodles from zucchini and cook another 2 minutes, stirring occasionally.
6. Put the shrimp back in the pan and mix well.
7. If necessary, add salt and pepper, garnish with parmesan and chopped parsley (optional) and serve immediately.

Calories: 404. Fat: 28 g. Protein: 32 g. Carbs: 5

Chicken Breasts in a Garlic-Cream Sauce

Prep. time: 10 minutes / Cook time: 25 minutes / Serves 4

For chicken: 2 Chicken breasts 1 tbsp. Lemon juice 1/4 tsp. Chili powder 1 tsp. Fresh grated ginger 1 Minced garlic ½ tsp. Coriander powder ½ tsp. Turmeric 1 oz. Butter

For the sauce: 4 oz. Heavy cream 3 tbsp. Crushed tomatoes 4 fl. oz. Chicken broth 1 Onion, diced 1 Garlic clove, minced 1/4 tsp. Chili powder 1 tsp. Fresh grated ginger 1/4 tsp. Cinnamon

1. Cut the chicken breasts into small pieces, then mix them in a bowl with lemon juice, chili powder, grated ginger, chopped garlic, coriander powder, turmeric, salt and pepper.
2. Heat 2 tablespoons of butter in a frying pan over medium heat, then add the onions and garlic, and simmer for 2 minutes or until fragrant.
3. Add chicken pieces and cook for 4-5 minutes. When the chicken is white, add heavy cream, chicken broth, chopped tomatoes, seasonings and mix well. Bring to a boil, then reduce the heat to minimum, cover and simmer for 6-7 minutes.
4. If you like sauce thicker - remove the lid and simmer it to the desired consistency.
5. Serve with steamed broccoli or any other low-carb product to your taste.

Calories: 319. Fat: 21 g. Protein: 27 g. Carbs: 3.9

Salmon Fillet with Cream Sauce

Prep. time: 10 minutes / Cook time: 15 minutes / Serves 3

2 tbsp. Olive oil 3 Salmon fillets 2 Garlic cloves, minced 1 cup Heavy whipped cream 1 oz. Cream cheese

2 tbsp. Capers 1 tbsp. Lemon juice 2 tsp. Fresh dill 2 tbsp. Parmesan cheese, grated

1. Place a large frying pan over medium heat and heat the olive oil. Once the pan is hot, add the salmon fillet, frying each side for about five minutes.
2. As soon as the salmon is cooked, remove it from the pan and set aside.
3. In the same pan, roast the chopped garlic over medium heat to a flavorful state.
4. Add heavy cream, cream cheese, lemon juice and capers.
5. Bring the mixture to a light boil, stirring often to thicken.
6. As soon as the sauce begins to thicken, put the salmon back in the pan and cover it with creamy sauce.
7. Reduce heat to medium-low - just to warm the fillet.
8. Garnish with fresh dill and grated Parmesan cheese.

Calories: 494. Fat: 31 g. Protein: 53 g. Carbs: 2.5

Beef Casserole with Cabbage and Cheese

Prep. time: 15 minutes / Cook time: 30 minutes / Serves 8

2 lb. Cauliflower 8 oz. Softened cream cheese 1 lb. Ground beef ½ Onion, diced 1 tbsp. Worcestershire Sauce 1 cup Shredded cracklings

1 Big egg 2 cup Cheddar cheese, grated 5 oz. Bacon Salt and pepper, to taste Extra side dish: chopped onion

1. Cut the bacon, and then fry it in a hot frying pan. Put it on a paper towel to absorb excess fat. Remove most of the fat from the pan, you will need only a few tablespoons.
2. Fry the onions in bacon fat until it is golden brown.
3. Add ground beef and fry well. Add the Worcestershire sauce and, if necessary, seasonings. Transfer the mixture to a large bowl.
4. In a separate bowl, mix the cabbage and cream cheese, then whisk everything together using a hand mixer or blender. The consistency of everything should be like mashed potatoes. If necessary, add seasoning.
5. Add chopped bacon and egg to beef mixture and mix well.
6. Place the ground beef on the bottom of the baking dish, and put the cauliflower puree on top.
7. Sprinkle casserole with chopped cheddar cheese and bacon.
8. Bake at 400 °F for 30 minutes.
9. If you want, sprinkle the finished dish with chopped onion.

Calories: 443. Fat: 35 g. Protein: 24 g. Carbs: 5.4

Creamy Spinach

Prep. time: 10 minutes / Cook time: 20 minutes / Serves 4

2 tbsp. Butter 2 tbsp. Olive oil 1 Onion, diced 2 Garlic cloves, minced

9 oz. Fresh spinach 2 fl. oz. Cream cheese 2 fl. oz. Heavy cream

1. Heat the cream and olive oil in a frying pan at medium-high temperature.
2. Add garlic and onions, and stir continuously for 2-3 minutes until soft.
3. Add the spinach (handful at a time) and fry until it withers. Put in a fine strainer and squeeze the liquid.
4. Return the spinach to the pan, season with pepper and salt, and add the heavy cream. Cook until bubbles in the cream.
5. Mix with cream cheese until it is completely melted, and the mixture is thick and bubbly. Remove from heat and serve.

Calories: 277. Fat: 21 g. Protein: 9 g. Carbs: 7

Fried Cod with Tomato Sauce

Prep. time: 10 minutes / Cook time: 20 minutes / Serves 4

A fish: 1 lb. (4 fillets) Cod 1 tbsp. Butter 1 tbsp. Olive oil Salt and pepper, to taste

Tomato sauce: 3 Large egg yolks 3 tbsp. Warm water 8 oz. Butter 2 tbsp. Tomato paste 2 tbsp. Fresh lemon juice

A fish:

1. Season the fillets on both sides. Note that the salt must be put at the last minute, before cooking, so as not to burn the fish.
2. Pour olive oil over the bottom of the anti-grate pan and turn on medium heat. Add butter. When

they begin to sizzle, add cod fillet and fry for two or three minutes, then turn it over to the other side.
3. Tilt the pan, collect the oil with a spoon and dip the fish in it. Continue cooking for another two or three minutes.

Tomato sauce:

1. Melt the butter.
2. Boil egg yolks and warm water (1 tablespoon of water for each egg yolk) for two minutes until thick and creamy.
3. Once the yolks have reached the desired consistency, remove them from the heat. Begin to beat them, slowly pouring in the butter. Beat until smooth.
4. Season with salt and pepper. You can also add herbs if you want.
5. Add tomato paste and mix.
6. Add lemon juice and adjust the consistency with a little warm water to slightly dilute the sauce.

Calories: 589. Fat: 56 g. Protein: 20 g. Carbs: 2

Braised Beef in Orange Sauce

Prep. time: 10 minutes / Cook time: 90 minutes / Serves 6

2 lb. Beef 3 cups Beef broth 3 tbsp. Coconut oil 1 Onion Peel and juice of 1 orange 2 tbsp. Apple vinegar 1 tbsp. Fresh thyme

2½ tsp. Garlic, chopped 2 tsp. Ground cinnamon 2 tsp. Erythritol 1 tsp. Soy sauce Rosemary, sage, bay leaf, salt, pepper, to taste

1. Cut vegetables and meat into cubes. Squeeze orange juice and rub it in zest.
2. Heat coconut oil in a cast iron skillet.
3. Add seasoned meat (salt + pepper) to the pan in batches. Do not overfill the pan.
4. Fry it until brown and remove from the pan.
5. As soon as your beef is ready, add vegetables to the pan. Cook for 1-2 minutes.
6. Add orange juice and then put all the other ingredients in the pan, with the exception of rosemary, sage and thyme.
7. Cook for 30 seconds, and then add all other ingredients.
8. Stew for 3 hours.
9. Open the pan and add the remaining spices. Let it cook for 1-2 hours.

Calories: 337. Fat: 14 g. Protein:42 g. Carbs: 5

Meatloaf

Prep. time: 10 minutes / Cook time: 60 minutes / Serves 8

1 lb. Ground beef ½ tsp. Garlic powder ½ tsp. Cumin 6 slices Cheddar cheese

2 oz. Sliced onions 2 oz. Green onions, chopped ½ cup Spinach ¼ cup Mushrooms

1. Mix the meat with salt, pepper, garlic and cumin. Put the stuffing in the form, leaving in the middle a place for the filling.
2. Put cheese on the bottom of the roll.
3. Add onions, spinach and mushrooms.
4. Use the remaining meat to cover the top with spinach and mushrooms as a lid.
5. Bake at 370 °F for one hour.

Calories: 248. Fat: 21 g. Protein: 15 g. Carbs: 2

Keto Chili

Prep. time: 10 minutes / Cook time: 30 minutes / Serves 6

2 lb. Young beef 8 oz. Spinach 1 cup Tomato sauce 2 oz. Parmesan cheese 2 Green bell peppers 1 Onion

1 tbsp. Olive oil 1 tbsp. Cumin 1½ tbsp. Chili powder 2 tsp. Cayenne pepper 1 tsp. Garlic powder Salt and pepper, to taste

1. Slice the onions and peppers. Then season with salt and pepper, and simmer in olive oil at medium high temperature, stirring occasionally. After the vegetables are ready, reduce the heat to minimum.
2. Fry the beef until brown. Season with salt, pepper and spices.
3. Once the beef is fried, add the spinach. Cook for 2-3 minutes, then mix well.
4. Add tomato sauce, mix well, then reduce the heat to medium-low and cook for 10 minutes.

5. Add Parmesan cheese and mix everything together. Then add the vegetables and mix again. Cook for a few minutes.

Calories: 404. Fat: 27 g. Protein: 31 g. Carbs: 5

Beef Croquettes with Sausage and Cheese

Prep. time: 10 minutes / Cook time: 30 minutes / Serves 12

1 lb. Minced beef 1 Chorizo sausage 1 cup Cheddar cheese 8 fl. oz. Tomato sauce

3 oz. Shredded pork skins 2 Large eggs 1 tsp. Cumin 1 tsp. Chili

1. Preheat oven to 380 °F degrees.
2. Cut the sausage into small pieces and mix well with the beef.
3. Add pork skins, spices, cheese and eggs.
4. Mix everything together until you can form the meatballs.
5. Place them on a baking sheet with a baking sheet.
6. Bake in the oven for 30-35 minutes.
7. Top with tomato sauce.

Calories: 142. Fat: 12 g. Protein: 7 g. Carbs: 1

Eggplant with Bacon

Prep. time: 10 minutes / Cook time: 20 minutes / Serves

1 lb. Bacon 1 lb. Eggplant 1 cup Heavy whipped cream 2 tbsp. Butter 2 Garlic cloves, grated

1 tbsp. White wine 1 tbsp. Lemon juice 1 cup Parmesan cheese, shredded

1. Slice the bacon and fry it in a large frying pan over medium heat.
2. When the bacon is crispy, pull it out of the pan and place it on a paper towel. Save all the fat.
3. Peel and slice the eggplant. Cook it in bacon fat until it softens.
4. As cooking progresses, the eggplant will absorb all the fat. Clean the center of the place and pour 2 tablespoons of oil into it. Stir everything so that the eggplants are covered in melted butter, then add the grated garlic.
5. Pour a cup of heavy whipped cream into the pan. Then add white wine and lemon juice.
6. Add a cup of shredded Parmesan cheese and mix.
7. Mix everything with about half the bacon.
8. Serve with the remaining bacon, laid out on top. You can also chop fresh basil from above.

Calories: 564. Fat: 51 g. Protein: 16 g. Carbs: 6

DESERTS

Cheesecake Keto-Cupcakes

Prep. time: 10 minutes / Cook time: 15 minutes / Serves 12

4 oz. Almond flour 2 oz. Butter, melted 8 fl. oz. Soft cream cheese

2 Eggs 6 oz. Granulated keto sweetener 1 tsp. Vanilla extract

1. Heat the oven to 350 °F degrees. Lay out the parchment 12 molds for muffins.
2. Mix together the almond flour and butter, then spread the mixture with a spoon over the forms and slightly push it inside.
3. Mix cream cheese, eggs, sweetener and vanilla extract with a mixer until smooth. Spread the spoon on top of the dough in the tins.
4. Bake in a preheated oven for 15 to 17 minutes.
5. Before serving, cupcakes should stand in the refrigerator for about 8 hours.

Calories: 204. Fat: 21 g. Protein: 4.9 g. Carbs: 2

Chocolates with Berries

Prep. time: 10 minutes / Cook time: 15 minutes / Serves 12

4 tbsp. Solid coconut oil 2 tbsp. Cocoa powder 1 tbsp. Erythritol or xylitol 1 tbsp. Liquid coconut oil

2 tbsp. Cocoa butter 1 cup Fresh berries mix Optional: grated unsweetened coconut or raw chopped nuts

1. Add solid coconut oil, cocoa butter, liquid coconut oil, salt, cocoa powder and sweetener to taste in a saucepan, then stir over low heat until completely dissolved.
2. Pour the chocolate mixture into the silicone tray for at least 12 forms. Sprinkle berries evenly (along with any other additives, if used).
3. Place the tray in the fridge for about 15 minutes.

4. Store leftovers in a refrigerator in a closed container.

Calories: 61. Fat: 6 g. Protein: 1 g. Carbs: 2

Keto Cookies with Raspberry Jam

Prep. time: 10 minutes / Cook time: 15 minutes / Serves 12

2 cup Almond flour 1/4 tsp Xanthan gum ½ tsp. Baking powder 4 oz. Soft butter 2 oz. Erythritol or other ketofriendly sweetener

1 tsp. Vanilla extract 1 Egg 3 tbsp. Raspberry jam / sugar free jam

1. Preheat the oven to 370 °F degrees and place a baking sheet with parchment paper.
2. Mix flour, xanthan gum, baking powder and salt in a small bowl. Put aside.
3. In a separate bowl, beat the butter and sweetener until the mass becomes airy.
4. Add egg and vanilla extract.
5. Add the flour mixture and mix well.
6. Divide the dough into 12 balls and place on the prepared baking sheet.
7. Click on the center of each ball to make a cookie. In the center of each place 1/2 tsp. of jam.
8. Bake cookies for 10–12 minutes, until the edges are light golden brown.
9. Allow to cool until the jam hardens.

Calories: 168. Fat: 16 g. Protein: 4 g. Carbs: 2

Chocolate Brownie in a Mug

Prep. time: 5 minutes / Cook time: 10 minutes / Serves 12

1 Big egg 2 tbsp. Almond flour ½ tsp. Baking powder 2 tbsp. Unsweetened cocoa powder

1 tbsp. Butter or coconut oil ½ tsp. Vanilla extract 1 tbsp. Stevia or keto-friendly sweetener of your choice

1. Oil one large cup or two small shapes. Put aside.
2. Add all ingredients to a small bowl and mix with a small whisk until smooth.
3. Pour the dough into the prepared form and place in the microwave for about 1 minute (two servings) or 75 seconds per serving in a mug.

Calories: 140. Fat: 9 g. Protein: 11 g. Carbs: 3

Lemon Blueberry Keto-Cakes

Prep. time: 10 minutes / Cook time: 20 minutes / Serves 12

Dough: 4 Eggs 3/4 cup Fatty coconut milk 1 tsp. Pure vanilla extract ½ cup Coconut flour 1½ tbsp. Xylitol 1 tsp. Baking powder ½ tsp. Xanthan gum 1/8 tsp. Pink Himalayan salt

3 tbsp. Herbal unsalted butter, melted 3/4 cup Fresh blueberries

Lemon icing: 1 Lemon, juice and zest 5 tbsp. Powdered (non-granular) stevia or xylitol

1. Preheat the oven to 370 °F degrees.

2. In a large bowl, mix the eggs, coconut milk and vanilla.
3. Add coconut flour, xylitol, baking powder, xanthan gum and salt, and beat well. Add melted butter and mix again.
4. Carefully add fresh blueberries.
5. Fill 12 cupcakes with dough, about half.
6. Place a baking tray with forms on the central grid of the oven and bake for about 20 minutes.
7. Remove from oven and cool.
8. Mix lemon juice with powdered sweetener and pour each cupcake with a small amount of icing. Garnish with fresh lemon peel.

Calories: 136. Fat: 7 g. Protein: 9 g. Carbs: 6

Chocolate Keto Fudge

Prep. time: 5 minutes / Cook time: 10 minutes / Serves 12

½ cup Almond oil ½ cup Coconut oil 2 oz. Unsweetened cocoa powder

3 tbsp. Keto sweetener 1 tsp. Vanilla extract 2 oz. Walnuts (optional)

1. Add coconut and almond oil, and cocoa powder in a blender, and beat until smooth.
2. Add vanilla, sweetener and salt. If desired, add walnuts or other ingredients to your taste.
3. Pour the mixture into a baking dish lined with parchment paper. Put it in the fridge until it is completely cool, then pull it out and cut it into 16 small squares.

Note: You can try to add the following toppings: Low carb chocolate crumb Some peanut butter Cream cheese Sea salt A few drops of peppermint oil

Calories: 137. Fat: 13 g. Protein: 3 g. Carbs: 2

Chocolate and Nutty Smoothies

Cooking time: 5 minutes/prep. time: 5 minutes/Serves 2

1 tbsp. Nutella 1 banana

½ cup Milk 2 oz. Pecans

1. Cut the banana into cuts, include some milk and a tablespoon of chocolate glue and pecans (6–8 pieces).
2. For 1–2 minutes, prepared to smooth with chocolate chips.

* Nutella can be supplanted with a large portion of a liquefied chocolate bar. From nuts, you can utilize hazelnuts.

Calories: 351. Fat: 23 g. Protein: 8 g. Carbs: 33

Keto Taco

Cooking Time: 10 minutes/prep. time: 20 minutes/Serves 3

Need to begin the day surprising? Morning keto is such an astonishing beginning to a lovely day. Light and magnificent with a lot of brilliant hues and feelings.

8 oz. Mozzarella cheddar, destroyed; 6 Eggs, enormous 2 tbsp. Spread

3 Bacon stripes ½ Avocado 1 oz. Cheddar, destroyed Pepper and salt to taste

1. Warmth a grill to 375 °F. Put the foil on a preparing sheet and spread the bacon on it. Cook it for 15-20 minutes.
2. While bacon is cooked, put 3 oz. of mozzarella in a spotless dish and cook cheddar over medium warmth.
3. Trust that the cheddar will cook around the edges (around 2-3 minutes).
4. Utilize a couple of tongs and a wooden spoon to make a cheddar shell for tacos.
5. Do likewise with the remainder of your cheddar.
6. Cook the eggs in the oil, mixing sporadically. Season with salt and pepper.
7. Spot 33% of the eggs, avocado and bacon in each solidified taco packaging.
8. Sprinkle with cheddar. Include hot sauce and cilantro whenever wanted.

Calories: 444. Fat: 36 g. Protein: 26 g. Carbs: 2.3

Keto Omelet with Goat Cheese and Spinach

Cooking time: 5 minutes/prep. time: 10 minutes/Serves 1

3 Large eggs 1 Medium green onion 1 oz. Goat cheddar ¼ Onion

2 tbsp. Spread 2 cups Spinach 2 tbsp. Overwhelming cream Salt and pepper to taste

1. Cut the onion into long strips and fry it in oil until caramelized. Add the spinach to the container and fry a bit.
2. Expel the vegetables from the container — blend 3 huge eggs, cream, salt and pepper together.
3. Empty the egg blend into the container and cook on medium warmth.
4. When the part of the omelette start to boil, include a spoonful of spinach and onions to 1/2 omelette. Sprinkle with hacked goat cheddar.
5. At the point when the highest point of the omelette is prepared, you can serve. On the off chance that you like, enliven with onions on top.

Calories: 621. Fat: 55 g. Protein: 37 g. Carbs: 4.8

Chicken and Cheese Quesadilla

Cooking time: 10 minutes/prep. time: 15 minutes/Serves 4

For tablets: 6 Eggs 4 oz. Coconut flour 6 oz. Overwhelming cream ½ tsp. Thickener Pink salt and pepper 1 tbsp. Olive oil for broilin

For the quesadilla: 4 oz. Cheddar destroyed 8 oz. Chicken bosom cooked and destroyed 1 tbsp. Parsley, hacked (discretionary)

1. Blend in a bowl every one of the ingredients for the cakes, whisk well and let the batter represent 8-10 minutes.

2. Warmth the oil in a griddle over medium warmth and fry the tortillas for 2-3 minutes on each side or until cooked. Put aside to cool.
3. Warmth, a spotless frying pan over medium warmth, put one tortilla, sprinkle with cheddar, spread with a top and hold up until the cheddar starts to dissolve. At that point include slashed chicken meat, more cheddar and covered with a subsequent level cake.

At the point when the cheddar has softened, expel the quesadilla from the container, cut into four cuts and sprinkle with crisp parsley before serving (discretionary).

NOTE: For best outcomes, use ground coconut flour. This will help with the surface, and you can make more slender cakes. A thickener will help make the tortilla stable and versatile. You can substitute fat cream with unsweetened almond milk. You can likewise decrease the number of eggs and include additional egg white. Be that as it may, you should test and modify the measure of flour used to acquire the ideal consistency.

Calories: 382. Fat: 31 g. Protein: 23 g. Carbs: 2.3

Vegan Scramble

Cooking time: 5 minutes/prep. time: 15 minutes/Serves 5

The formula is anything but difficult to plan yet delectable avocados, tomatoes and cheeses will lift your spirits and invigorate for extraordinary deeds.

1 lb. Tofu cheddar 3 tbsp. Avocado oil 2 tbsp. Slashed onion 1½ tbsp. Nourishment yeast ½ tsp. Garlic powder

½ tsp. Turmeric ½ tsp. Salt 1 cup Spinach 3 Grape tomatoes 3 oz. Vegetarian Cheddar Cheese

1. Envelop the tofu by a few layers of paper or fabric towels, and delicately press some water. Set aside.
2. In a skillet over medium warmth, fry the cleaved onion in 1/3 tbsp. Avocado spread until onion is delicate and translucent
3. Spot the tofu in the dish and mix well with a fork.
4. Pour the rest of the oil and sprinkle with dry flavouring.
5. Fry the tofu over medium warmth, blending once in a while until the majority of the fluid has dissipated.
6. Include the spinach, dice the tomatoes and cheddar, and cook for a moment or until the spinach has blurred and the cheddar has softened.
7. Serve hot and store scraps in the cooler for a limit of three days.

Calories: 211. Fat: 17.6 g. Protein: 10 g. Carbs: 4.7

Burger with Guacamole and Egg

Cooking time: 5 minutes/prep. time: 10 minutes/Serves 1

Here and there in the morning, you truly need a delicious burger with different flavours. Thusly, I have arranged for this superb formula. Succulent meat, bright guacamole, an egg and 10 minutes is all you have to make the most of your most loved keto burgher. Everybody around will need the equivalent.

5 oz. Ground hamburger 4 Bacon, cuts 3 oz. Guacamole 1 Egg

1 tbsp. Olive oil (for fricasseeing) ½ tsp. Italian flavouring Salt and pepper to taste

1. In a little bowl, blend ground hamburger with Italian flavouring, salt and pepper. Structure a little patty.
2. Put on a cutting board 4 portions of bacon across, cutlet on top, and afterwards fold bacon over it.
3. Warmth 1/2 tablespoons of olive oil in a griddle over medium warmth, include the cutlet in bacon and fry 3 minutes (or more, contingent upon thickness) on each side
4. Include the staying 1/2 tablespoons of oil to the dish and fry the egg, with the fluid yolk inside.
5. Put guacamole, a seared egg on a cutlet, and, if vital, season with salt and pepper. Cut down the middle and serve right away.

Calories: 443. Fat: 33 g. Protein: 32.5 g. Carbs: 2.4

Stuffed Avocado

Cooking time: 5 minutes/prep. time: 10 minutes/Serves 1

1 Avocado hollowed and cut down the middle 1 tbsp. Spread, salted 3 Large eggs

3 cuts of bacon, cut into little pieces Salt and dark pepper, to taste

1. Wipe out the greater part of the avocado mash, leaving about 1.5 cm around.
2. Spot a huge skillet over low warmth and include margarine. While the spread is dissolving, break the eggs into a bowl and whisk them, including a touch of salt and pepper.
3. Spot bacon on one side of the container and fry for two or three minutes. On the opposite side, pour the egg blend and mix them routinely.
4. Eggs and bacon ought to be readied 5 minutes in the wake of adding eggs to the dish. In the event that you find that the eggs are cooked a little before the bacon, expel the fried eggs and spot them in a bowl.
5. Blend the bacon and fried eggs together, and afterwards fill the avocado parts with the blend.

Calories: 500. Fat: 40 g. Protein: 25 g. Carbs: 11

Omelette with Mushrooms and Goat Cheese

Cooking time: 5 minutes/prep. time: 10 minutes/Serves 1

3 Large eggs 2 tsp. Overwhelming cream 3 oz. Cleaved mushrooms 1 tsp. Olive oil

2 oz. Disintegrated goat cheddar Seasoning to taste Green onions for trimming

1. Warmth olive oil in a dish. Fry the mushrooms until delicate, about. 4 minutes.
2. While the mushrooms are being cooked, beat the eggs with overwhelming cream and a modest quantity of flavouring.
3. Pour the egg blend over the mushrooms and cook for around 2-3 minutes.

4. Include goat cheddar. Overlay the omelette into equal parts and keep cooking until the cheddar begins to soften.
5. Present with spring onions or another side dish to your taste.

Calories: 515. Fat: 39.5 g. Protein: 21 g. Carbs: 4.2

Fat Bombs

Neapolitan Fatty Bombs

Cooking time: 10 minutes/prep. time: 15 minutes/Serves 24

½ cup Butter ½ cup Coconut oil ½ cup Sour cream ½ cup Cream cheddar 2 tbsp. Erythritol

25 drops Liquid stevia 2 tbsp. Cocoa powder 1 tsp. Vanilla concentrate 2 medium strawberries

1. Utilizing a blender, blend every one of the ingredients (aside from cocoa powder, vanilla and strawberry) in a bowl.
2. Partition the blend between 3 dishes. Add cocoa powder to one, vanilla to another, and strawberries to third.
3. Empty the chocolate blend into the shape and spot in the cooler for 30 minutes. Rehash the procedure with vanilla and strawberry layers.
4. Presently put all stop for in any event 60 minutes.

Calories: 102. Fat: 11 g. Protein: 1 g. Carbs: 0.

Chocolate-Coconut Fat Bombs with Almonds

Cooking time: 5 minutes/prep. time: 15 minutes/Serves 12

1 cup Coconut chips 3 tbsp. Fat coconut milk 3 tbsp. Coconut oil (softened) ½ tsp. Vanilla concentrate

4 oz. Chocolate chips, no sugar A spot of salt 2 oz. Keto-accommodating sugar 24 Almond, pieces

1. Put 2 tablespoons of softened coconut oil, coconut milk, sugar, coconut chips, vanilla concentrate and salt in a little bowl.
2. Separation the blend into 12 servings and spot them on a preparing sheet with material paper. Put in the cooler for 5 minutes, at that point put on each fat bomb 1-2 things almonds.
3. Liquefy the chocolate chips together with 2 teaspoons of coconut oil in the microwave.
4. Expel the bombs from the cooler, pour every one of the chocolate blend and cool.

Calories: 92. Fat: 9 g. Protein: 2 g. Carbs: 1.5

Spicy Fat Bombs

Cooking time: 5 minutes/prep. time: 15 minutes/Serves 12

6 MCT powder scoops 10 Liquid stevia, drops 1 tsp. Turmeric 1 tbsp. Dark sesame seeds

Squeeze Chinese 5 Spice Blend A touch of dark pepper ½ tsp. Cinnamon 2½ fl. oz. Warm water

1. Blend all the dry ingredients in a little bowl.
2. Include warm water and blend until smooth.

3. Spread the blend equally more than 12 silicone moulds, around 1 tbsp. L on each.
4. Put in the refrigerator, so the fat bombs are all around solidified. Continuously keep them solidified, else they will rapidly soften.

Calories: 81. Fat: 8 g. Protein: 1 g. Carbs: 1.5

Espresso Fat Bombs

Cooking time: 5 minutes/prep. time: 30 minutes/Serves 12

4 oz. Margarine 2 oz. Ghee spread (liquefied) 2 oz. Substantial cream 1 tbsp. Milk to your taste Double coffee

2 oz. Keto-accommodating sugar of your decision 1 tsp. Vanilla concentrate A spot of salt

1. Add all ingredients to a little nourishment processor and whip at rapid until vaporous.
2. Add sugar to taste.
3. Fill shape and refrigerate for 30 minutes (or more in the event that you wish)

Calories: 61. Fat: 5 g. Protein: 1 g. Carbs: 1

Almond Coconut Fat Bombs

Cooking time: 5 minutes/prep. time: 20 minutes/Serves 10

2 fl. oz. Almond oil 2 fl. oz Coconut oil

2 tbsp. Cocoa powder 2 fl. oz Erythritol, to your taste

1. Blend almond and coconut oil in a microwave dish.
2. Warmth the blend in the microwave for 30-45 seconds and blend until a homogeneous mass. Include erythritol and cocoa powder, and blend to finish the blend.
3. Empty the mass into scaled-down cupcake forms and refrigerate in the icebox.

Calories: 89. Fat: 9.3 g. Protein: 1.5 g. Carbs: 1

Pumpkin Fat Spice Bombs

Cooking time: 5 minutes/prep. time: 10 minutes/Serves 9

8 oz. Crude cashews 4 oz. Crude macadamia nuts 4 oz. Coconut chips 3 fl. oz. Pumpkin puree

2 tbsp. MCT oils 2 tsp. Cinnamon, ground 2 tsp. Ginger, ground Neutral oil (avocado oil)

1. Put every one of the ingredients in a nourishment processor and blend to frame a mixture.
2. Delicately oil your hands with nonpartisan oil, for example, avocado oil. Utilizing a spoon, take about 3.5 - 4 oz. of the hitter into softly oiled hands and structure a ball. Defer and rehash the procedure (around 9 "bombs" altogether).
3. Brighten fat bombs with appetizing coconut chips.
4. Such greasy bombs can be eaten promptly, or put away in an icebox/cooler.

Calories: 217. Fat: 19 g. Protein: 5 g. Carbs: 5

Cheddar Fat Bombs in Bacon

Cooking time: 5 minutes/prep. time: 20 minutes/Serves 20

8 oz. Mozzarella cheddar 4 tbsp. Almond flour 4 tbsp. Spread, dissolved 3 tbsp. Psyllium powder 1 Egg Salt, to taste

1 tsp. Dark pepper 1/8 tsp. Garlic powder 1/8 tsp. Onion powder 20 Bacon, cuts 1 cup oil or fat (for searing)

1. Microwave, a large portion of the cheddar for 45-60 seconds or until it, softens and ends up clingy.
2. Warmth the margarine in the microwave for 15-20 seconds until totally softened, at that point blend it with cheddar and egg.
3. Include psyllium husks, almond flour and flavours. Blend again and spread out the mixture square shape.
4. Fill the square shape with the remainder of the cheddar and overlap it into equal parts (on a level plane), at that point down the middle (vertically).
5. Trim the edges and structure into a square shape. Cut 20 square pieces.
6. Wrap each bit of mixture with a bit of bacon, utilizing toothpicks to secure it.
7. Put each piece in bubbling oil and cook for 1-3 minutes.

Calories: 93. Fat: 8 g. Protein: 5 g. Carbs: 1Servings of mixed greens

Vegetable Salad with Bacon and Cheese

Cooking time: 5 minutes/prep. time: 10 minutes/Serves 6

4 oz. Lettuce 3 oz. Spinach 2 oz. Wavy cabbage 6 cuts of cooked bacon 12 pcs. grape tomato

1 Avocado stripped and cut 2 oz. Blue cheddar 3 tbsp. Harsh cream 2 ½ tbsp. Mayonnaise

1. In a little bowl, blend the harsh cream and mayonnaise.
2. Blend with a large portion of the blue cheddar and put in a safe spot.
3. In an enormous plate of mixed greens bowl, blend the rest of the ingredients.
4. Spread the serving of mixed greens into segments and spot the blue cheddar dressing on top.

Calories: 183. Fat: 16 g. Protein: 6.5 g. Carbs: 2.5

A plate of mixed greens with Chicken Breast and Greens

Cooking time: 10 minutes/prep. time: 30 minutes/Serves 2

2 tbsp. Pesto sauce 2 fl. oz. Balsamic vinegar 1 tsp. Olive oil 6 oz. Chicken bosom 4 cup Spring greens

1 oz. New mozzarella ¼ Avocado, diced 6 Cherry tomatoes 1 tbsp. New basil for adornment

1. Set up the marinade by blending pesto, balsamic vinegar and olive oil
2. Put in a safe spot a segment of the marinade for the serving of mixed greens, and pour the staying chicken bosom. Refrigerate marinate for in any event 20 minutes.
3. Take the serving of mixed greens. Start with greens, at that point layered with crisp mozzarella, avocado and tomatoes.

4. When the chicken is salted, heat the medium-sized iron, and afterwards include a little olive oil.
5. Fry each side of the bosom for 7-10 minutes.
6. Cut the chicken bosom and spot on the recently arranged serving of mixed greens.
7. Pour the staying balsamic pesto and include some cleaved new basil.

Calories: 306. Fat: 16 g. Protein: 25 g. Carbs: 6.5

Salmon Salad

Cooking time: 5 minutes/prep. time: 10 minutes/Serves 2

2 Sheets of lettuce 6 leaves, Fresh basil, finely hacked ½ tsp. Garlic powder 1 tsp. Lemon juice

4 tbsp. Mayonnaise 5 oz. Salmon 1 oz. Red onion, hacked ½ Avocado, diced 2 tbsp. Parmesan cheddar, diced

1. Wash well and clean the lettuce leaves - they will fill in as plates.
2. Blend lemon juice hacked basil and garlic powder.
3. Include mayonnaise and blend well. Put in a safe spot.
4. Fill each "plate" of lettuce with half of the finely slashed salmon, and after that avocado and onion rings.
5. Top with equitably mastermind the mayonnaise (prior around 2 tablespoons for every serving), at that point place the parmesan 3D squares.

Calories: 373. Fat: 31 g. Protein: 19.6 g. Carbs: 2.5

Basic Cabbage and Egg Keto Salad

Cooking time: 10 minutes/prep. time: 10 minutes/Serves 6

1 lb. Cauliflower flowers 4 oz. Keto mayonnaise 1 tsp. Yellow mustard 1½ tsp. Crisp dill Ground dark pepper and salt, to taste 2 oz. Finely slashed dill

1 Celery stalk finely slashed 2 oz. Red onion slashed 1 tbsp. Salted keto cucumber, cleaved 6 Hard-bubbled eggs, hacked Paprika, for enhancement

1. Pour some water (about 2.5 cm) into an enormous pan, put 1 tsp. of salt and heat to the point of boiling. Include cauliflower and cook until prepared, from 8 to 10 minutes. Channel and put aside in an enormous bowl.
2. In a little bowl, blend mayonnaise, mustard, dill, a spot of salt and pepper. Put in a safe spot.
3. Pulverize 4 eggs and add to the cauliflower bowl. Cut the staying two eggs.
4. Include cured cucumber, celery, 1/4 teaspoon salt, pepper and red onion. Add every one of the ingredients to the cauliflower and shake tenderly.
5. Embellishment with the staying hacked eggs and sprinkle with paprika.

Calories: 222. Fat: 20 g. Protein: 8 g. Carbs: 2

Light Pea and Green Onion Salad

Cooking time: 5 minutes/Cook time: 10 minutes/Serves

2 oz. Pea 2 tsp. Green onions ½ tsp. Soy sauce 2 tsp. Olive oil

½ tsp. Apple vinegar ½ tsp. Sesame oil ½ tsp. Sesame seeds Garlic powder, to taste

1. Cut the green onions and peas corner to corner.
2. Blend the cleaved vegetables with the rest of the ingredients and blend. Spread and refrigerate for 2 hours.
3. Present with your preferred primary course - flame-broiled chicken, shrimps, salmon, and so on.

Calories: 136. Fat: 14 g. Protein: 2.5 g. Carbs:

Keto-Salsa with Avocado and Shrimps

Cooking time: 10 minutes/Cook time: 10 minutes/Serves 4

8 oz. Stripped crude shrimp 1 tbsp. Olive oil 1 Lemon (juice) 1 Avocado, diced 1 Tomato, diced

1 Cucumber, diced 1/4 Onion, diced 2 oz. Cilantro, hacked Salt and dark pepper, to taste.

1. Season the shrimp with salt and pepper. Put the dish on medium-high heat and pour olive oil. When the oil has heated up, include the shrimp and fry one side for 2-3 minutes, at that point go to the next.
2. Expel the shrimps from the skillet and put them on a cutting board. Cut and move to a huge bowl.

3. Crush the marinade lemon juice into the bowl. Blend well and let represent some time.
4. Include bits of avocado, tomatoes and cucumbers to the bowl.
5. Blend with cleaved onion and cilantro. Combine well all.

Calories: 283. Fat: 18.8 g. Protein: 18 g. Carbs: 6.2

Keto Salad Taco

Cooking time: 10 minutes/prep. time: 20 minutes/Serves 4

1 lb. Ground hamburger from grass-bolstered meat 1 tsp. Ground cumin ½ tsp. Bean stew powder 1 tbsp. Garlic powder ½ tbsp. Pepper and Paprika Salt, to taste 4 cups Roman lettuce

1 Tomato 4 oz. Cheddar 4 oz. Cilantro 1 Avocado 4 oz. Most loved salsa 2 little limes 1 cup Cucumber, cut

1. Warmth a huge skillet over medium warmth and pour in some coconut oil. Include ground hamburger and all seasonings.
2. Blend well and fry until darker. Expel from warmth and cool somewhat.
3. Blend roman lettuce, vegetables, cheddar and slashed avocado. Top with meat, salsa and a liberal segment of lime juice. Blend everything admirably.

Calories: 430. Fat: 31 g. Protein: 29 g. Carbs:

Bites

Fast Keto Bread

Cooking time: 5 minutes/prep. time: 10 minutes/Serves 10

2 tbsp. Almond flour ½ tbsp. Coconut flour 1/4 tsp. Preparing powder 1 Egg

½ tbsp. Ghee or spread 1 tbsp. Unsweetened milk of your choice

1. Blend all ingredients in a little bowl and speed until smooth.
2. Oil a glass bowl or microwave dish with spread, ghee or coconut oil.
3. Empty the batter into a form and spot in the microwave at high temperature for 90 seconds.
4. Cut and pour softened margarine as wanted.

Calories: 45. Fat: 20 g. Protein: 7 g. Carbs: 3

Note: If you don't have a microwave, have a go at singing the batter in a modest quantity of spread/coconut oil or ghee. A similar cooking time, the equivalent

Vitality Keto Bars with Nuts and Seeds

Cooking time: 10 minutes/prep. time: 25 minutes/Serves 8

2 tbsp. Margarine or coconut oil 2 fl. oz. Without sugar 1 tsp. Vanilla concentrate 8 oz. Almond, hacked 8 oz. Crude macadamia nuts (finely hacked) 4 oz. Pumpkin seed

2 tbsp. Hemp seed 1-2 tsp. Keto sugar (if important) 4 oz. Low sugar chocolate chips ½ tsp. Coconut or spread, or ghee oil

1. Preheat the stove to 350 °F degrees and spread out a preparing dish with material paper. Put every one of the nuts and seeds in a huge bowl, and blend.
2. Soften spread or coconut oil with vanilla concentrate and syrup in a little pan over low heat.
3. Pour the hot blend over the nuts and seeds, and shake well. On the off chance that essential, include keto sugar (erythritol, stevia, and so forth.)
4. Empty the subsequent mass into the readied heating dish.
5. Heat for around 22-25 minutes until the top turns brilliant dark coloured. Allow the blend to cool for in any event 45 minutes.
6. Soften the chocolate and 1/2 tsp of coconut oil in the microwave or on the stove. Pour a blend of heated nuts and seeds.
7. Put in the cooler for 10-15 minutes. Expel from the shape and cut into 8 pieces.

Calories: 303. Fat: 29 g. Protein: 8 g. Carbs: 4

Low-Carb Flax Bread

Cooking time: 10 minutes/prep. time: 15 minutes/Serves 8

1 oz. Almond flour 1½ Flaxseed 1 tsp. Heating powder Salt, to taste ½ tsp. Vinegar

4 drops liquid stevia 3 oz. Crude whisked egg 1 fl. oz. Coconut oil or margarine (liquefied)

1. Combine all the dry ingredients, at that point, blend the wet ones.
2. Blend dry ingredients with wet ones.
3. Spread the mixture into a daintily oiled structure.
4. Heat at 350 °F degrees for 8–10 minutes.

Calories: 35. Fat: 42 g. Protein: 14 g. Carbs: 6

Keto Mini Pizza

Cooking time: 5 minutes/prep. time: 15 minutes/Serves 4

1 oz. Keto mayonnaise 1 tbsp. Crude eggs 2 tsp. Coconut oil softened 2 tsp. Almond flour

1 tsp. Coconut flour ½ tsp. Psyllium powder A spot of preparing powder and heating pop

1. Warmth the broiler to 400 °F degrees.
2. Blend every one of the ingredients well to shape a batter. Ensure there are no irregularities in it.
3. Leave the mixture to represent around 5 minutes.
4. Partition the batter into 3-4 little balls, about 2.5 cm in width.
5. Spread out a heating sheet with material paper. Put batter balls on the material and press down on them to make little pizzas.
6. Put the stuffing on the crude batter and prepare for 7-9 minutes.

Calories: 112. Fat: 28 g. Protein: 4 g. Carbs: 2

Prepared Eggs with Ham and Asparagus

Cooking time: 5 minutes/: 15 minutes/Serves

6 Eggs 6 cuts (around 4 oz.) Italian ham 8 oz. Asparagus

A couple of sprigs of new marjoram 1 tbsp. Spread or ghee

1. Warmth the stove to 350 °F degrees.
2. Oil a biscuit plate.
3. Lay the ham down and around the gap in order to cover the base and sides.
4. Include a couple of twigs of marjoram.
5. Empty 1 egg into each structure.
6. Put in the broiler and prepare 10 - 12 minutes until cooked.
7. Destroy out and allow to cool for a couple of minutes.
8. Steam the asparagus, at that point season it with margarine
9. Put every one of the ingredients on a plate and appreciate.

Calories: 424. Fat: 33 g. Protein: 30 g. Carbs: 2.5

Eggplant Keto Chips

Cooking time: 5 minutes/prep. time: 20 minutes/Serves 4

2 fl. oz. Olive oil 1 Large eggplant (daintily cut) Sal and pepper to taste 1 tsp. Garlic powder

½ tsp. Dry basil ½ tsp. Dried oregano 2 tbsp. Parmesan cheddar

1. Preheat broiler to 350 °F degrees.
2. Include 1/4 cup olive oil and dried flavours to a little bowl. Roll the cut eggplant in oil and flavours, and spot it on a heating sheet.

3. Heat for around 15-20 minutes, until the chips are equally singed. Turn them over multiple times during cooking.
4. Expel from the broiler and sprinkle with Parmesan cheddar (discretionary)

Calories: 60. Fat: 5 g. Protein: 2 g. Carbs: 1

Cheddar Keto Sticks

Cooking time: 5 minutes/prep. time: 15 minutes/Serves 3

3 Mozzarella cheddar sticks (cut down the middle) 4 oz. Almond flour 1 tbsp. Italian flavouring blends 2 tbsp. Ground parmesan cheddar

1 Big egg Salt, to taste 2 tbsp. Coconut oil 1 tbsp. Cleaved parsley

1. Put the cheddar in the cooler medium-term with the goal that it solidifies.
2. At that point add coconut oil to a medium measured cast iron skillet and warmth it over low to medium warmth.
3. Break the egg into a shallow bowl and whisk well. In a different bowl, blend the almond flour, parmesan cheddar and seasonings.
4. Move cheddar sticks in an egg, at that point dry breading. Put on a wire rack and prepare until brilliant dark coloured on all sides for around 12 minutes.
5. Spot chopsticks on paper towels to absorb the oil.
6. Present with low-carb marinara sauce and parsley (discretionary).

Calories: 436. Fat: 39 g. Protein: 20 g. Carbs: 5

LUNCH

Chicken Keto Nuggets

Cooking time: 15 minutes/prep. time: 6 hours/Serves 4

1 oz. Whipped egg whites 1 oz. Chicken bosom cooked and minced ½ oz. Coconut flour ½ tsp. Preparing powder

1 fl. oz. Olive oil ½ oz. Dissolved margarine 1 oz. Greasy 40% cream Salt, pepper, a touch of garlic powder, discretionary

1. Blend destroyed chicken with coconut flour, preparing powder and flavouring. The blend should look dry.
2. Include spread and blend once more. Include whipped egg whites and blend until smooth.
3. Empty olive oil into a little non-stick dish. Spread the chicken-egg blend in little pieces and fry for around 1 moment on each side.
4. Present with whipped cream, weakened with water, similar to "milk".

Calories: 136. Fat: 41 g. Protein: 9 g. Carbs: 2

Champignon Keto Burger

Cooking time: 5 minutes/prep. time: 15 minutes/Serves 4

Ground meat ½ tsp. Garlic powder

½ tsp. Onion powder ½ tsp. Worcestershire Sauce 1 cheddar, cut 1 Slice of tomato 2 oz. Blended greens or arugula 1 tbsp. Low-sugar ketchup

1. Put the mushroom tops in a bowl or shallow plate, and include olive oil, balsamic vinegar and a large portion of the salt and pepper; marinate for at any rate 30 minutes.
2. Cook the bacon in a griddle over medium warmth until fresh, turning two or multiple times to broil each side equally. Put in a safe spot.
3. Preheat the stove and turn on the barbecue work (270 °F degrees). Blend in a bowl ground hamburger, garlic and onion powder, Worcestershire sauce, and the staying salt and pepper. Structure of the patties for burgers.
4. Put the tops of champignons and cutlets on the barbecue, and cook for around 3-4 minutes on each side until they are delicate. Finally, put the cheddar on the cutlets, so it liquefies.
5. Gather the cheeseburger with bacon and the remainder of the stuffing between the mushroom tops.

Calories: 771. Fat: 67 g. Protein: 37 g. Carbs: 4

Feeding Beef Soup

Cooking time: 10 minutes/prep. time: 30 minutes/Serves

1 lb. Ground meat 5 Slices of bacon 1 tbsp. Olive oil 1 tbsp. Minced garlic 1 cup Chopped celery 1½ cup Bone stock.

1 cup Shredded cheddar 2 fl. oz. Fat whipped cream 2 tsp. Psyllium powder 4 oz. Destroyed cheddar ½ oz. Hacked green onions ½ cup Sour cream

1. Fry the bacon over medium warmth, at that point place it on paper towels to evacuate abundance fat. At that point, smash it into pieces.
2. At that point fry the ground meat over medium warmth. Subsequent to cooking, channel the fat and move the minced meat to a bowl.
3. In a similar container, soften spread over medium warmth. Include hacked garlic and fry until fragrant.
4. Include the celery and cook until somewhat relaxed, around 5 minutes.
5. Put the ground meat in the skillet. Include hamburger soup, cheddar, rich whipped cream, sautéed celery with garlic, bacon, salt and pepper. Cook for 20 minutes, mixing periodically.
6. To acquire the ideal thickness, include psyllium powder.
7. Fill parts and include a side dish as cheddar, green onions and harsh cream (discretionary).

Calories: 349. Fat: 27 g. Protein: 23 g. Carb

Keto Cheeseburger with Bacon

Cooking time: 10 minutes/prep. time: 30 minutes/Serves 2

For the mixture: 8 oz. Mozzarella destroyed 4 oz. Almond flour 1 tbsp. Cream cheddar

For the filling: 5 oz. Ground hamburger 1 Slice of cheddar, cut into quarters

1 tsp. Mustard 4 Bacon, cuts 1 Whisked egg 1 tsp. Sesame 1 tsp. Olive oil Salad Leaves for Garnish (Optional)

1. Preheat broiler to 420 °F degrees.
2. Blend mozzarella, almond flour and cream cheddar in a bowl. Warmth the blend in the microwave for 1 moment, blend and re-set in the microwave for 1 moment.
3. Structure two patties from ground meat. Put on the cutting board 4 pieces of bacon transversely, cutlet on top, at that point cheddar cuts, the subsequent cutlet, and after that wrap all the bacon.
4. Roll the mixture between 2 sheets of material paper. Evacuate the top sheet and spot mustard in the focal point of the mixture. On top, put the patty in bacon and wrap the batter.
5. Put the burger on the stove, cover with beaten egg, sprinkle with sesame seeds and prepare for 15-20 minutes or until brilliant darker.
6. Take out and present with sheets of greens.

Calories: 411. Fat: 32 g. Protein: 27 g. Carbs: 3

Hot Keto Soup with Mushrooms

Cooking time: 10 minutes/prep. time: 30 minutes/Serves 4

1 tbsp. Olive oil 1 Onion (daintily cut) 1 tbsp. Crisp ground ginger 3 Garlic, cloves (finely cleaved) 1 tsp. Chile 1 tbsp. Fish sauce

2 fl. oz. Soy sauce 2 fl. oz. Rice vinegar 4 oz. Mushrooms (daintily cut) 4 Hard bubbled eggs 2-3 parcels of shirataki noodles 5 cup Bone stock

1. Empty oil into a huge pan and put on medium warmth. Include the onion and cook for 2-3 minutes until delicate.
2. Add the rest of the ingredients to the dish (with the exception of eggs and noodles) — Cook over low heat for 20-30 minutes.
3. Expel the noodles from the bundle and wash well under virus water.
4. Add flavouring to the soup and blend with noodles.
5. Empty the soup into parts. Include hard-bubbled eggs, cleaved chicken or hamburger, cilantro, sesame seeds, slashed green onions and stew sauce (all discretionary).

Calories: 103. Fat: 13 g. Protein: 12 g. Carbs: 7

Greek Keto Moussaka

Prep. time: 10 minutes/Cook time: 30 minutes/Serves

For the filling: ½ Chopped eggplant 10 oz. You have minced chicken 3 tbsp. Marinara sauce 1 Minced garlic ½ Chopped onion 1 tsp. Dried oregano 1 tsp. Paprika

½ tsp. Ground cinnamon 2 tbsp. Olive oil

For the sauce: 3 tbsp. Overwhelming cream 3 tbsp. Cream cheddar 3 oz. Squashed cheddar 1 Minced garlic

1. Spread out a foil heating sheet. Cut the eggplants, put them on a preparing sheet and pour olive oil.

Prepare the eggplants for 5 minutes or until brilliant dark coloured.
2. Warmth olive oil in a griddle, include hacked onion, cleaved garlic and fry until delicate. Include cleaved chicken and seasonings, and fry until the meat is cooked. Include the marinara sauce, blend and cook for an additional 3 minutes.
3. Blend a large portion of the squashed cheddar, cream cheddar, substantial cream, garlic and salt in a pot, and cook on low heat until the cheddar is liquefied and the sauce turns out to be thick and uniform.
4. Preheat broiler to 400 °F degrees. Spot the bits of singed eggplant on a preparing sheet, top the chicken blend, pour the sauce, sprinkle with the rest of the cheddar and heat for 20 minutes.
5. Give the dish a chance to represent 5 minutes before serving. May be presented with a green plate of mixed greens or greens.

Calories: 358. Fat: 29 g. Protein: 20 g. Carbs: 4

Almond Pancakes with Shrimp and Cheese

Prep. time: 10 minutes/Cook time: 10 minutes/Serves 8

1 lb. Shrimp cooked and cleaved 2 oz. Almond flour 1 Whisked egg 2 oz. Mozzarella, destroyed

3 tbsp. Parmesan cheddar, ground 1 tbsp. Crisp dill hacked 1½ tbsp. Olive or coconut oil, for fricasseeing Salt and pepper, to taste

1. Blend the shrimp, egg, almond flour, cheddar, dill and seasonings in a bowl and blend well until smooth.

2. Utilizing a tablespoon to shape flapjacks. The size of each relies upon your taste.
3. Warmth the oil in a dish over medium warmth and fry hotcakes for 3-4 minutes on each side or until cooked.
4. Put on a plate and present with herbs and aioli, or some other sauce of your decision.

Calories: 364. Fat: 21 g. Protein: 41 g. Carbs: 2

DINNER

Heated Halibut Cheese Breaded

Cooking time: 10 minutes/prep. time: 15 minutes/Serves 6

2 lb. Halibut (around 6 filets) 1 tbsp. Margarine 3 tbsp. Ground parmesan cheddar 1 tbsp. Bread scraps

2 tsp. Garlic powder 1 tbsp. Dried parsley Salt and pepper, to taste

1. Preheat the broiler to 400 °F degrees. Blend all ingredients completely in a bowl, with the exception of the plate.
2. Dry the fish with the paper towel and spot each piece on a lubed buttered material plate.
3. Spread the cheddar blend into bits of fish with the goal that it covers its top.
4. Prepare the fish for 10-12 minutes (turn the heating plate in any event once).
5. Increment heat for 2–3 minutes until the top is brilliant dark coloured. Check preparation with a fork.

Calories: 330. Fat: 30 g. Protein: 13 g. Carbs: 2

Baked Chicken Legs

Prep. time: 10 minutes/Cook time: 25 minutes/Serves 2

2 Whole chicken legs 4 fl. oz. Greasy Greek yoghurt 2 tbsp. Olive oil ½ tsp. Cumin ½ tsp. Turmeric ½ tsp. Coriander 1/4 tsp. Cardamom

½ tsp. Cayenne pepper 1 tsp. Paprika Pinch of Nutmeg 1 Minced garlic clove ½ tsp. Crisp ginger 2 tbsp. Lime juice Salt and pepper, to taste

1. Warmth olive oil in a little griddle over medium warmth. Include cumin, turmeric, coriander, cardamom, cayenne pepper, paprika and a touch of nutmeg. Warmth the flavours, at that point, expel from warmth and cool.
2. Blend in a bowl yoghurt with spiced oil, lime juice, ginger, hacked garlic, salt and pepper.
3. Make 3-4 profound cuts on every leg and empty hot yoghurt into them. Spread and refrigerate for 6 hours.
4. Grease up the rack for fricasseeing olive oil and spot on a heating sheet. Put the chicken on the rack and fry for 5 minutes on each side.
5. Set the stove to 360 °F degrees and keep cooking for 25 minutes.
6. Present with cauliflower rice.

Calories: 372. Fat: 28 g. Protein: 30 g. Carbs: 2

Prepared Eggplant with Cheese

Prep. time: 15 minutes/Cook time: an hour/Serves 4

1 Large eggplant, cut 1 Big egg ½ cup Parmesan cheddar, ground ¼ cup Pork batter

½ tbsp. Italian flavouring 1 cup low-sugar tomato sauce ½ cup Mozzarella, destroyed 4 tbsp. Spread

1. Preheat stove to 400 °F degrees. Put the cut eggplant on a heating sheet fixed with a paper towel and sprinkle with salt on the two sides. Let represent in any event 30 minutes with the goal that all the water leaves the eggplant.
2. Blend the slashed pork cracklings, parmesan cheddar and Italian flavouring in a shallow dish. Put in a safe spot.
3. In a different little plate, beat an egg.
4. Soften the spread and oil the heating dish with it.
5. Plunge each bit of eggplant in a beaten egg, and afterwards in a blend of parmesan and cracklings, covering each side with morsels.
6. Spot the eggplants in a heating dish and prepare for 20 minutes. Turn the eggplant cuts over and heat for an additional 20 minutes or until brilliant dark coloured.
7. Top with tomato sauce and sprinkle with slashed mozzarella.
8. Return the shape to the broiler for an additional 5 minutes, or until the cheddar has liquefied.

Calories: 376. Fat: 28 g. Protein: 19 g. Carbs: 7

Shrimp and Zucchini with Alfredo Sauce

Cooking time: 5 minutes/prep. time: 15 minutes/Serves 6

8 oz. Shrimp stripped 2 tbsp. Margarine ½ tsp Minced garlic 1 tbsp. Crisp lemon juice

2 Zucchini 2 oz. Substantial cream 3 oz. Parmesan cheddar Salt and pepper to taste

1. Utilize the scoop to make zucchini noodles.
2. Warmth the margarine in a griddle, include the slashed garlic, red pepper and fry for 1 moment, blending continually.
3. Include shrimp and stew for around 3 minutes. Include salt and pepper, expel from the dish and put in a safe spot.
4. In a similar dish (with shrimp juice), include substantial cream, lemon juice, parmesan, and cook for 2 minutes.
5. Include the noodles from zucchini and cook an additional 2 minutes, mixing once in a while.
6. Set the shrimp back in the container and blend well.
7. In the event that vital, include salt and pepper, decorate with parmesan and slashed parsley (discretionary) and serve right away.

Calories: 404. Fat: 28 g. Protein: 32 g. Carbs: 5

Chicken Breasts in a Garlic-Cream Sauce

Cooking time: 10 minutes/Cook time: 25 minutes/Serves 4

For the chicken: 2 Chicken bosoms 1 tbsp. Lemon juice 1/4 tsp. Bean stew powder 1 tsp. Crisp ground ginger 1 Minced garlic ½ tsp. Coriander powder ½ tsp. Turmeric 1 oz. Margarine

For the sauce: 4 oz. Substantial cream 3 tbsp. Squashed tomatoes 4 fl. oz. Chicken soup 1 Onion, diced 1 Garlic clove, minced 1/4 tsp. Stew powder 1 tsp. Crisp ground ginger 1/4 tsp. Cinnamon

1. Cut the chicken bosoms into little pieces, at that point blend them in a bowl with lemon juice, bean stew powder, ground ginger, hacked garlic, coriander powder, turmeric, salt and pepper.
2. Warmth 2 tablespoons of spread in a griddle over medium warmth, at that point, include the onions and garlic, and stew for 2 minutes or until fragrant.
3. Include chicken pieces and cook for 4-5 minutes. At the point when the chicken is white, include substantial cream, chicken soup, slashed tomatoes, seasonings and blend well. Boil it, at that point lessen the warmth to least, spread and stew for 6-7 minutes.
4. If you like the sauce thicker - expel the top and stew it to the ideal consistency.
5. Present with steamed broccoli or some other low-carb item to your taste.

Calories: 319. Fat: 21 g. Protein: 27 g. Carbs: 3.9

Salmon Filet with Cream Sauce

Cooking time: 10 minutes/Cook time: 15 minutes/Serves 3

2 tbsp. Olive oil 3 Salmon filets 2 Garlic cloves, minced 1 cup heavy whipped cream 1 oz. Cream cheddar

2 tbsp. Tricks 1 tbsp. Lemon juice 2 tsp. Crisp dill 2 tbsp. Parmesan cheddar, ground

1. Spot a huge skillet over medium warmth and warmth the olive oil. When the skillet is hot, include the salmon filet, fricasseeing each side for around five minutes.
2. When the salmon is cooked, expel it from the container and put in a safe spot.
3. In a similar container, cook the cleaved garlic over medium warmth to a delightful state.
4. Include substantial cream, cream cheddar, lemon squeeze and escapades.
5. Carry the blend to a light bubble, regularly mixing to thicken.
6. When the sauce starts to thicken, set the salmon back in the container and spread it with velvety sauce.
7. Decrease warmth to medium-low - to warm the filet
8. Embellishment with crisp dill and ground Parmesan cheddar.

Calories: 494. Fat: 31 g. Protein: 53 g. Carbs: 2.5

Meat Casserole with Cabbage and Cheese

Cooking time: 15 minutes/Cook time: 30 minutes/Serves 8

2 lb. Cauliflower 8 oz. Mollified cream cheddar 1 lb. Ground hamburger ½ Onion, diced 1 tbsp. Worcestershire Sauce 1 cup Shredded cracklings

1 Big egg 2 cup cheddar, ground 5 oz. Bacon Salt and pepper, to taste Extra side dish: cleaved onion

1. Cut the bacon, and after that fry it in a hot skillet. Put it on a paper towel to ingest overabundance fat. Expel a large portion of the fat from the dish, and you will require just a couple of tablespoons.
2. Fry the onions in bacon fat until it is brilliant darker.
3. Include ground hamburger and fry well. Include the Worcestershire sauce and, if essential, seasonings. Move the blend to a huge bowl.
4. In a different bowl, blend the cabbage and cream cheddar, at that point whisk everything together utilizing a hand blender or blender. The consistency of everything ought to resemble pureed potatoes in the event that fundamental, including flavouring.
5. Add cleaved bacon and egg to hamburger blend and blend well.
6. Spot the ground hamburger on the base of the heating dish, and put the cauliflower puree on top.
7. Sprinkle meal with slashed cheddar and bacon.
8. Heat at 400 °F for 30 minutes.
9. On the off chance that you need, sprinkle the completed dish with slashed onion

Calories: 443. Fat: 35 g. Protein: 24 g. Carbs: 5.4

Rich Spinach

Cooking time: 10 minutes/Cooking time: 20 minutes/Serves 4

2 tbsp. Margarine 2 tbsp. Olive oil 1 Onion, diced 2 Garlic cloves, minced

9 oz. Crisp spinach 2 fl. oz. Cream cheddar 2 fl. oz. Substantial cream

1. Warmth the cream and olive oil in a griddle at medium-high temperature.
2. Include garlic and onions, and mix ceaselessly for 2-3 minutes until delicate.
3. Include the spinach (bunch at once) and fry until it wilts. Put in a fine strainer and press the fluid.
4. Return the spinach to the dish, season with pepper and salt, and include the substantial cream. Cook until air pockets in the cream.
5. Blend with cream cheddar until it is totally dissolved, and the blend is thick and bubbly. Expel from warmth and serve.

Calories: 277. Fat: 21 g. Protein: 9 g. Carbs: 7

Seared Cod with Tomato Sauce

Cooking time: 10 minutes/Cook time: 20 minutes/Serves 4

A fish: 1 lb. (4 filets) Cod 1 tbsp. Spread 1 tbsp. Olive oil Salt and pepper, to taste

Tomato sauce: 3 Large egg yolks 3 tbsp. Warm water 8 oz. Spread 2 tbsp. Tomato glue 2 tbsp. Crisp lemon juice

A fish:

1. Season the filets on the two sides. Note that the salt must be placed ultimately, before cooking, so as not to consume the fish.

2. Pour olive oil over the base of the counter mesh skillet and turn on medium warmth. Include spread. When they start to sizzle, include cod filet and fry for a few minutes, at that point give it to the opposite side.
3. Tilt the dish, gather the oil with a spoon and plunge the fish in it. Keep cooking for another a few minutes.

Tomato sauce:

1. Dissolve the margarine.
2. Bubble egg yolks and warm water (1 tablespoon of water for each egg yolk) for two minutes until thick and smooth.
3. When the yolks have arrived at the ideal consistency, expel them from the warmth. Start to beat them, slowly pouring in the spread. Beat until smooth.
4. Season with salt and pepper. You can likewise include herbs on the off chance that you need.
5. Include tomato glue and blend.
6. Include lemon squeeze and alter the consistency with a little warm water to marginally weaken the sauce.

Calories: 589. Fat: 56 g. Protein: 20 g. Carbs: 2

Braised Beef in Orange Sauce

Prep. time: 10 minutes/Cook time: an hour and a half/Serves 6

2 lb. Meat 3 cups Beef soup 3 tbsp. Coconut oil 1 Onion Peel and squeeze of 1 orange 2 tbsp. Apple vinegar 1 tbsp. Crisp thyme

2½ tsp. Garlic hacked 2 tsp. Ground cinnamon 2 tsp. Erythritol 1 tsp. Soy sauce Rosemary, wise, cove leaf, salt, pepper, to taste

1. Cut vegetables and meat into 3D shapes. Press squeezed orange and rub it in pizzazz.
2. Warmth coconut oil in a cast-iron skillet.
3. Include prepared meat (salt + pepper) to the container in clumps. Try not to pack the skillet.
4. Fry it until dark-coloured and expel from the skillet
5. When your hamburger is prepared, add vegetables to the container — Cook for 1-2 minutes.
6. Include squeezed orange and after that put the various ingredients in the skillet, except for rosemary, sage and thyme.
7. Cook for 30 seconds, and after that include every single other ingredient.
8. Stew for 3 hours.
9. Open the dish and include the rest of the flavours. Give it a chance to cook for 1-2 hours.

Calories: 337. Fat: 14 g. Protein:42 g. Carbs: 5

Meatloaf

Prep. time: 10 minutes/Cook time: an hour/Serves

1 lb. Ground hamburger ½ tsp. Garlic powder ½ tsp. Cumin 6 cuts cheddar

1. 2 oz. Cut onions 2 oz. Green onions slashed ½ cup Spinach ¼ cup Mushrooms.
2. Blend the meat with salt, pepper, garlic and cumin. Put the stuffing in the structure, leaving in the centre a spot for the filling.
3. Put cheddar on the base of the roll.
4. Include onions, spinach and mushrooms.
5. Utilize the rest of the meat to cover the top with spinach and mushrooms as a top.
6. Prepare at 370 °F for 60 minutes.

Calories: 248. Fat: 21 g. Protein: 15 g. Carbs: 2

Keto Chili

Cooking time: 10 minutes/Cook time: 30 minutes/Serves 6

2 lb. Youthful meat 8 oz. Spinach 1 cup Tomato sauce 2 oz. Parmesan cheddar 2 Green ringer peppers 1 Onion

1 tbsp. Olive oil 1 tbsp. Cumin 1½ tbsp. Stew powder 2 tsp. Cayenne pepper 1 tsp. Garlic powder Salt and pepper, to taste

1. Cut the onions and peppers. Add salt and pepper, and stew in olive oil at medium-high temperature, mixing at times. After the vegetables are prepared, diminish the warmth to least.
2. Fry the meat until darker. Season with salt, pepper and flavours.
3. When the meat is singed, include the spinach. Cook for 2-3 minutes, at that point, blend well.

4. Include tomato sauce, blend well, at that point lessen the warmth to medium-low and cook for 10 minutes.
5. Gather Parmesan cheddar and blend everything into a single unit. At that point include the vegetables and blend once more — Cook for a couple of minutes.

Calories: 404. Fat: 27 g. Protein: 31 g. Carbs: 5

Hamburger Croquettes with Sausage and Cheese

Cooking time: 10 minutes/Cook time: 30 minutes/Serves 12

1 lb. Minced hamburger 1 Chorizo frankfurter 1 cup cheddar 8 fl. oz. Tomato sauce

3 oz. Destroyed pork skins 2 Large eggs 1 tsp. Cumin 1 tsp. Bean stew

1. Preheat broiler to 380 °F degrees.
2. Cut the frankfurter into little pieces and blend well with the hamburger.
3. Include pork skins, flavors, cheddar and eggs.
4. Combine everything until you can shape the meatballs
5. Spot them on a heating sheet with a preparing sheet.
6. Heat in the stove for 30-35 minutes.
7. Top with tomato sauce.

Calories: 142. Fat: 12 g. Protein: 7 g. Carbs: 1

Eggplant with Bacon

Cooking time: 10 minutes/Cook time: 20 minutes/Serves

1 lb. Bacon 1 lb. Eggplant 1 cup Heavy whipped cream 2 tbsp. Margarine 2 Garlic cloves, ground

1 tbsp. White wine 1 tbsp. Lemon juice 1 cup Parmesan cheddar, destroyed.

1. Cut the bacon and fry it in an enormous skillet over medium warmth.
2. At the point when the bacon is firm, haul it out of the dish and spot it on a paper towel. Spare all the fat.
3. Strip and cut the eggplant. Cook it in bacon fat until it relaxes.
4. As for cooking advances, the eggplant will retain all the fat. Clean the focal point of the spot and empty 2 tablespoons of oil into it. Mix everything with the goal that the eggplants are canvassed in softened margarine, at that point include the ground garlic.
5. Pour a cup of the overwhelming whipped cream into the dish. At that point include white wine and lemon juice
6. Include a cup of destroyed Parmesan cheddar and blend.
7. Blend everything with about a large portion of the bacon.
8. Present with the rest of the bacon, spread out on top. You can likewise hack new basil from above.

Calories: 564. Fat: 51 g. Protein: 16 g. Carbs: 6

DESERTS

Cheesecake Keto-Cupcakes

Cooking time: 10 minutes/Cook time: 15 minutes/Serves 12

4 oz. Almond flour 2 oz. Spread, dissolved 8 fl. oz. Delicate cream cheddar

2 Eggs 6 oz. Granulated keto sugar 1 tsp. Vanilla concentrate

1. Warmth the stove to 350 °F degrees. Spread out the material 12 moulds for biscuits.
2. Combine the almond flour and margarine, at that point spread the blend with a spoon over the structures and somewhat drive it inside.
3. Blend cream cheddar, eggs, sugar and vanilla, concentrate with a blender until smooth. Spread the spoon over the batter in the tins
4. Heat in a preheated stove for 15 to 17 minutes.
5. Prior to serving, cupcakes should remain in the cooler for around 8 hours.

Calories: 204. Fat: 21 g. Protein: 4.9 g. Carbs: 2

Chocolates with Berries

Cooking time: 10 minutes/Cook time: 15 minutes/Serves 12

4 tbsp. Strong coconut oil 2 tbsp. Cocoa powder 1 tbsp. Erythritol or xylitol 1 tbsp. Fluid coconut oil

2 tbsp. Cocoa spread 1 cup Fresh berries blend Optional: ground unsweetened coconut or crude slashed nuts.

1. Include strong coconut oil, cocoa spread, fluid coconut oil, salt, cocoa powder and sugar to taste in a pot, at that point blend over low heat until totally broke up.
2. Empty the chocolate blend into the silicone plate for at any rate 12 structures. Sprinkle berries equally (alongside some other added substances, whenever utilized).
3. Spot the plate in the ice chest for around 15 minutes
4. Store scraps in a cooler in a shut compartment.

Calories: 61. Fat: 6 g. Protein: 1 g. Carbs: 2

Keto Cookies with Raspberry Jam

Cooking time: 10 minutes/Cook time: 15 minutes/Serves 12

2 cup Almond flour 1/4 tsp Xanthan gum ½ tsp. Heating powder 4 oz. Delicate margarine 2 oz. Erythritol or other keto-friendly sugar

1 tsp. Vanilla concentrate 1 Egg 3 tbsp. Raspberry jam/sugar free jam

1. Preheat the broiler to 370 °F degrees and spot a heating sheet with material paper.
2. Blend flour, thickener, preparing powder and salt in a little bowl. Set aside.
3. In a different bowl, beat the spread and sugar until the mass ends up breezy.
4. Include egg and vanilla concentrate.
5. Include the flour blend and blend well.
6. Gap the mixture into 12 balls and spot on the readied preparing sheet.

7. Snap-on the focal point of each ball to make a treat. In the focal point of each spot 1/2 tsp. of jam.
8. Heat treats for 10–12 minutes until the edges are light brilliant dark coloured.
9. Allow cooling until the jam solidifies.

Calories: 168. Fat: 16 g. Protein: 4 g. Carbs: 2

Chocolate Brownie in a Mug

Cooking time: 5 minutes/Cooking time: 10 minutes/Serves 12

1 Big egg 2 tbsp. Almond flour ½ tsp. Heating powder 2 tbsp. Unsweetened cocoa powder

1. 1 tbsp. Margarine or coconut oil ½ tsp. Vanilla concentrate 1 tbsp. Stevia or keto-accommodating sugar of your decision
2. Oil one enormous cup or two little shapes. Set aside.
3. Add all ingredients to a little bowl and blend with a little race until smooth.
4. Empty the mixture into the readied structure and spot in the microwave for around 1 moment (two servings) or 75 seconds for every serving in a mug.

Calories: 140. Fat: 9 g. Protein: 11 g. Carbs: 3

Lemon Blueberry Keto-Cakes

Cooking time: 10 minutes/prep. time: 20 minutes/Serves 12

Batter: 4 Eggs 3/4 cup Fatty coconut milk 1 tsp. Unadulterated vanilla concentrate ½ cup Coconut flour 1½ tbsp. Xylitol 1 tsp. Heating powder ½ tsp. Thickener 1/8 tsp. Pink Himalayan salt

3 tbsp. Homegrown unsalted spread, dissolved 3/4 cup Fresh blueberries

Lemon icing: 1 Lemon, squeeze and get-up-and-go 5 tbsp. Powdered (non-granular) stevia or xylitol

1. Preheat the stove to 370 °F degrees.
2. In a huge bowl, blend the eggs, coconut milk and vanilla.
3. Include coconut flour, xylitol, preparing powder, thickener and salt, and beat well. Include dissolved margarine and blend once more.
4. Cautiously include new blueberries
5. Fill 12 cupcakes with batter, about half.
6. Spot a preparing plate with structures on the focal network of the stove and heat for around 20 minutes.
7. Expel from stove and cool.
8. Blend lemon juice with powdered sugar and pour every cupcake with a limited quantity of icing — embellishment with the new lemon strip.

Calories: 136. Fat: 7 g. Protein: 9 g. Carbs: 6

Chocolate Keto Fudge

Cooking time: 5 minutes/prep. time: 10 minutes/Serves 12

½ cup Almond oil ½ cup Coconut oil 2 oz. Unsweetened cocoa powder

3 tbsp. Keto sugar 1 tsp. Vanilla concentrate 2 oz. Pecans (discretionary)

1. Include coconut and almond oil, and cocoa powder in a blender, and beat until smooth.
2. Include vanilla, sugar and salt. Whenever wanted, add pecans or different ingredients to your taste.
3. Empty the blend into a heating dish fixed with material paper. Put it in the ice chest until it is totally cool, at that point, haul it out and cut it into 16 little squares.

Note: You can attempt to include the following garnishes: Low carb chocolate morsel Some nutty spread Cream cheddar Sea salt A couple of drops of peppermint oil

Calories: 137. Fat: 13 g. Protein: 3 g. Carbs: 2

Cheesecake Mint

Cooking time: 10 minutes/Cook time: 15 minutes/Serves 6

1½ cup Almond flour 2½ cup Powdered erythritol 5 tbsp. Liquefied margarine 1 lb. Delicate cream cheddar

15 Whole mint leaves 2 fl. oz cup Heavy cream 6 oz — low-carb dark chocolate 1/4 tsp. Mint concentrate.

1. Preheat the broiler to 176 degrees.
2. Spot a square heating sheet with material paper.

3. In an enormous bowl, blend the almond flour and a large portion of some erythritol.
4. Empty the liquefied margarine into the bowl and blend the ingredients until the batter is shaped.
5. Put the mixture on a heating sheet and prepare for 8 minutes or until light dark-coloured.
6. Expel the container from the broiler and cool.
7. Make the filling, whipping cream cheddar and remaining erythritol with a blender until smooth.
8. Put mint leaves and overwhelming cream in a nourishment processor and mix until smooth.
9. Add the mint blend to the cream cheddar filling and blend well.
10. Put the stuffing on the batter in a heating sheet, at that point put it in the cooler for 3 hours.
11. Take out the cheesecake from the container, cut into 64 squares and set it back in the cooler
12. Liquefy the chocolate in the microwave, regularly blending, until it ends up fluid.
13. Include mint concentrate, at that point plunge or sprinkle each bit of cheesecake with mint chocolate and let it cool.

Calories: 121. Fat: 12 g. Protein: 3 g. Carbs: 2

STAPLES

Handcrafted Keto Mayo

Cooking time: 5 minutes/prep. time: 10 minutes/Serves 12

6 fl. oz. Olive oil 4 fl. oz. Coconut oil 1 Egg 2 Egg yolks

1 tsp. Dijon mustard Pinch of salt and smoked paprika 3 drops Liquid Stevia.

1. Start by adding oils to the blender bowl to gauge them. Ensure your coconut oil isn't hot.
2. Include every other ingredient.
3. Start blending without lifting the blender.
4. Keep blending by holding the blender at the base of the compartment.
5. Move the blender all over until the mayonnaise is completely emulsified.
6. Put the mayonnaise in a glass container with a cover and spot in the cooler. In the event that you are utilizing whey, leave on a rack for 7 hours, at that point refrigerate.

NOTE: If you don't have a plunge blender, put all ingredients, with the exception of margarine, in your blender or nourishment processor, and turn it on. Carefully and slowly start, including oil. As the mayonnaise emulsifies, you can begin including oil somewhat quicker, until you arrive at a constant flow.

(1 tbsp.) Calories: 130. Fat: 14 g. Protein: 1 g. Carbs: 0.5

Handcrafted Sambal Sauce

Cooking time: 5 minutes/prep. time: 30 minutes/Serves 10

1 Onion 2 tsp. Stew peppers dried 3 tbsp. Low-sugar ketchup 2 tbsp. Coconut oil Salt, to taste

1. Cut the onion and blend until smooth. Put in a safe spot.

2. Straightforward chillies and expel the seeds. Heat up the peppers for around 30 minutes or until delicate. At that point, transform the pepper into a glue.
3. In a warmed skillet, dissolve coconut oil. Add every one of the ingredients and blend completely.

(1 tbsp.) Calories: 36. Fat: 3 g. Protein: 0.5 g. Carbs: 1.5

Low Carb Ketchup

Time: 5 minutes/Cook time: 5 minutes/Serves 10

3/4 cup Tomato glue 2 tbsp. Apple juice vinegar 2 tsp. Keto sugar Pinch of salt

1 tsp. Garlic powder 3/4 tsp. Onion Pinch powder of Cayenne Pepper 1 cup Water

1. Add every one of the ingredients to a huge bowl and whisk well.
2. Change the salt and sugar to taste.

(1 tbsp.) Calories: 20. Fat: 0 g. Protein: 1 g. Carbs: 2

Dutch Keto Sauce

Cooking time: 5 minutes/Cook time: 5 minutes/Serves 10

6 Egg yolks 1 drop Worcestershire sauce 1 drop Low carb hot sauce 1 Lemon, juice

A squeeze of salt and ground dark pepper 8 oz. Margarine

NOTE: The way to progress is to ensure your margarine is hot enough to cook eggs gently. It is basic that you include the oil following expelling it from the microwave.

1. Put the initial 5 ingredients in a blender. Warmth the spread in the microwave (spread with a paper towel, so it doesn't sprinkle) for 2-3 minutes.
2. Set the blender to low speed and rapidly pour the oil through the highest point of the blender. Beat around 10-15 seconds until smooth.

Calories: 120. Fat: 12 g. Protein: 2 g. Carbs: 1

Tapenade Keto Sauce

Cooking time: 5 minutes/prep time: 5 minutes/Serves 8

1 cup Black olives in saline solution 1 oz. Tricks 4 fl. oz. Blend Olive and Avocado oils 2 Garlic, cloves

3 tbsp. Lemon juice 2 tsp. Apple juice vinegar 1 cup Fresh basil 1 cup Fresh parsley ½ tsp. Dark pepper

1. Put every one of the ingredients in a blender or nourishment processor, and beat at low speed until totally homogeneous.
2. Fill dishes and store in the cooler for as long as 1 week.

Calories: 134. Fat: 14 g. Protein: 1 g. Carbs: 2

Meat Keto Sauce

Cooking: 5 minutes/Cook time: 5 minutes/Serves 8

1 Shallot 4 Garlic, cloves ½ cup Cilantro ½ cup Parsley 1 Lemon juice

3 tbsp. Red wine vinegar 2 tsp. Squashed red pepper Pinch of salt and dark pepper ¼ cup Olive oil

1. Blend all ingredients with the exception of olive oil in a nourishment processor. Proceeding to beat, pour the oil through the highest point of a ceaseless stream.
2. Season to taste and include more oil and two or three tablespoons of water, if important, with the goal that the sauce is increasingly liquid.

Calories: 46. Fat: 4 g. Protein: 1 g. Carbs: 1

Speedy Pickled Keto Vegetables

Cooking time: 5 minutes/Cook time: 5 minutes/Serves 10

1½ cup Filtered water 1½ cup Apple juice vinegar 1½ tbsp. Pink Himalayan salt

Discretionary: 1/4 tsp. granulated stevia

Recommended vegetables for snappy pickling: 6 little entire carrots ½ Asparagus, with cut finishes ½ cup Thinly cut cucumber ½ cup Thinly cut red onion

1. seIn a little pot over medium warmth, blend every one of the ingredients for the brackish water. Warmth the fluid to a delicate bubble until the salt and sugar break down (around 2 minutes).
2. Spread the vegetables into the containers and cautiously fill them with saltwater. Allow the containers to cool, at that point close the covers and store in the icebox (as long as 2 months).

Calories: 10. Fat: 0.1 g. Protein: 0.1 g. Carbs: 2

Made in the USA
Coppell, TX
09 June 2021